D1719005

Zhao Xi-wu

Experience in Pattern Differentiation

Project Editor: Wang Li-zi
Copy Editor: Liu Li-xiang
Book & Cover Designer: Yin Yan
Typesetter: Wei Hong-bo

Masters of Chinese Medicine Series

Zhao Xi-wu
Experience in Pattern Differentiation

● Complied by
Xi Yuan Hospital of China Academy of Chinese Medical Science

Translated by
Li Zhao-guo (李照国), Ph.D. TCM,
Prof. of English, Shanghai Normal University
Wang La-ping (汪腊萍), M.S. English
Vice Prof. of English, Shanghai Normal University

Edited by
Barclay Calvert, MAOM

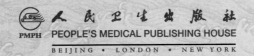

PMPH **PEOPLE'S MEDICAL PUBLISHING HOUSE**
BEIJING · LONDON · NEW YORK

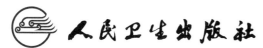

PMPH   PEOPLE'S MEDICAL PUBLISHING HOUSE

Website: http://www.pmph.com

Book Title: Masters of Chinese Medicine Series:
Zhao Xi-wu Experience in Pattern Differentiation
名老中医经验集系列：赵锡武医疗经验

Contact address: Bldg 3, 3 Qu, Fang Qun Yuan, Fang Zhuang, Beijing 100078, P.R. China, phone/fax: 86 10 6761 7315, E-mail: pmph@pmph.com

First published: 2008
ISBN: 978-7-117-10225-4/R·10226

Cataloguing in Publication Data:
A catalog record for this book is available from the CIP-Database China.

Printed in P. R. China

ISBN 978-7-117-10225-4

〖 Zhao Xi-wu，赵锡武 〗

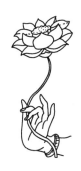

Zhao Xi-wu (1902-1980), professor and famous TCM expert, began studying Chinese medicine when he was 15. His expertise was treating various diseases of internal medicine, such as cardiovascular disease, diabetes, kidney disease and infantile apoplexy. He was the director of the Internal Medicine Department at Xi Yuan Hospital (affiliated hospital of the China Academy of TCM), the vice president of the China Academy of TCM, and the vice director of the China Association of TCM. His representative work is Zhao Xi-wu Experience in Pattern Differentiation (赵锡武医疗经验).

〖 Publisher's Foreword 〗

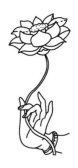

● *Yue Mei-zhong*, *Zhao Xi-wu*, *Shi Jin-mo*, and *Pu Fu-zhou* were among the number of China's famous traditional doctors who were not only thoroughly steeped in classical learning but were also diligent students of modern science. At a time when Western medicine was asserting greater influence in China, these doctors encouraged the perpetuation of Chinese medicine, yet also saw the usefulness of biomedicine's diagnostic and treatment advancements—they served as a link between the past and the future in the modern development of Chinese medicine. The books in this series were all written in the last years of the author's lives; in some cases right up to their deaths. Regardless of whether these works were written by the author himself, transmitted to another author, or compiled by their students, each one reflects the essence of its author's lifelong study and clinical experience.

● The doctors represented in this series are an exception to the traditional transmission of knowledge to a select few students. They sought to uplift Chinese medicine and share their knowledge so that more people could benefit from it.

● The case studies and theoretical knowledge provided in this series not only have high clinical value, but also offer a spark of creativity in a field that often finds comfort in platitudes. The medical essays are eloquent and explain the profound in simple terms, a rarely seen combination for the student of Chinese medicine and an invaluable guide for the practitioner.

● The works represented in the Masters of Chinese medicine series were first published by the People's Medical Publishing House from the 1960s to the 1980s; continuously well-received, they have sold many tens of thousands of copies. Out of print for some time, many are difficult to come by, and some are even collectors' items for students of Chinese medicine. The impact on the field of Chinese medicine left by these works cannot be overstated; they did much to promote the field of Chinese medicine as well as to raise its standards.

● Other than formatting changes, we have done our best to maintain the flavor of the original works so that the reader may appreciate them as when they were first published. Hence, alternate names for herbs, disease, and technical terms have been left unchanged. In keeping with this principle, medicinals which are currently illegal, such as *xī jiǎo* (Rhinoceros horn) and *hǔ gǔ* (Tiger bone) have been retained as in the original. It is the publisher's hope that practitioners will use the appropriate substitutes.

People's Medical Publishing House
Beijing, May, 2008

Foreword for First Edition

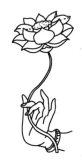

● The late professor Zhao Xi-wu (1902-1980) was the vice president of the China Academy of Traditional Chinese Medicine. He began studying TCM at an early age, and devoted 50 years to the study and practice of TCM. He is a renowned TCM expert who founded his own unique method of treating various obstinate diseases, often utilizing large dosages of medicinals.

● This book, based on the manuscripts of Professor Zhao and other relevant material, was compiled by his students, Guo Yu-ying, Zhang Wen-qu, An Bang-yi and Chen Ke-ji, and briefly summarizes the clinical experience of Professor Zhao in the treatment of various illnesses. Some of the manuscripts were provided by his other students, Yu Tian-xing, Li Xiang-guo and Wang Zhan-xi.

Xi Yuan Hospital of the China Academy of
Traditional Chinese Medicine
Beijing, 1979

China Academy of Traditional Chinese Medicine (CATCM)
(renamed as China Academy of Chinese Medical Science, CACMS, in 2007)

TABLE OF CONTENTS

CHAPTER 1   DIFFERENTIATION OF PATTERNS AND DIFFERENTIATION OF DISEASES 001

CHAPTER 2   PATHOGENESIS AND TREATMENT OF CORONARY HEART DISEASE.. 013

Understanding Coronary Heart Disease in Chinese Medicine 014

Causes of Coronary Heart Disease 017

Treatment of Coronary Heart Disease 018

Conclusion 024

CHAPTER 3   TREATMENT OF CHRONIC CARDIOPULMONARY DISEASE 027

Chinese Medicine Diagnosis 028

Treatment Based on Pattern Differentiation 029

Clinical Treatment 031

CHAPTER 4   TREATMENT OF MYOCARDITIS 035

CHAPTER 5   BRIEF COMMENTS ON SLOW PULSE..................... 043

CHAPTER 6   TREATMENT OF CONGESTIVE HEART FAILURE WITH *ZHĒN WŬ TĀNG* (TRUE WARRIOR DECOCTION) COMBINED WITH THE THREE METHODS USED TO TREAT EDEMA 047

CHAPTER 7   PATHOGENESIS AND TREATMENT OF ACUTE AND
CHRONIC NEPHRITIS 067
How Chinese Medicine Understands Nephritis 068
Treatment Principles... 070

CHAPTER 8   TREATMENT OF PYELONEPHRITIS 077

CHAPTER 9   TREATMENT OF DIABETES MELLITUS 081

CHAPTER 10   DISCUSSION ON SUPERFICIAL PATTERNS 085

CHAPTER 11   THERAPEUTIC METHODS FOR DEALING
WITH FEVERS... 087

CHAPTER 12   TREATMENT OF INFANTILE PNEUMONIA
PATTERN 095
On Pneumonia Pattern 096
On the Cause and Pathogenesis of the Disease 096
Pattern Differentiation and Diagnosis 097
Treatment Principles for Pneumonia 099

CHAPTER 13   TREATMENT OF COUGH AND DYSPNEA 107

Wind-cold and Wind-heat Types of Cough and Dyspnea 109

Chronic Cough and Dyspnea 111

Commonly Used Methods to Treat Cough and Dyspnea Based on

Differentiation of Phlegm 113

CHAPTER 14   TREATMENT OF PLEURAL DISEASES 117

CHAPTER 15   TREATMENT OF ULCER DISEASE 121

CHAPTER 16   TREATMENT OF DIARRHEA 127

CHAPTER 17   TREATMENT OF DYSENTERY.............................. 137

CHAPTER 18   TREATMENT OF MALARIA................................ 141

CHAPTER 19   TREATMENT OF POLIOMYELITIS 147

CHAPTER 20   TREATMENT OF EPILEPSY PATTERN 157

CHAPTER 21   TREATMENT OF TRIGEMINAL NEURALGIA........... 163

CHAPTER 22   TREATMENT OF *BǍI HÉ* (LILY DISEASE) 167

CHAPTER 23 TREATMENT OF NEURASTHENIA 173

CHAPTER 24 TREATMENT OF WIND STROKE 177

CHAPTER 25 EXPERIENCE IN USING *DÌ HUÁNG YĬN ZĬ*
(REHMANNIA DRINK) 183

CHAPTER 26 TREATMENT OF COLD HERNIA 191

CHAPTER 27 TREATMENT OF MALE STERILITY 195

CHAPTER 28 TREATMENT OF LUPUS ERYTHEMATOSUS............ 199

CHAPTER 29 PATHOGENESIS AND TREATMENT OF SKIN
DISEASES 213

CHAPTER 30 TREATMENT OF THREATENED MISCARRIAGE AND
FUNCTIONAL UTERINE BLEEDING WITH MODIFIED *HUÁNG TŬ
TĀNG* (YELLOW EARTH DECOCTION) 219

CHAPTER 31 TREATMENT OF AUDITORY VERTIGO
(MENIERE DISEASE) 223

CHAPTER 32 TREATMENT OF ARTHRITIS 229
    Active Stage 231

Inactive Stage 233

CHAPTER 33   COMMENTS ON *HÚ HUÒ* (BEHCET'S
SYNDROME) 239

INDEX BY DISEASE NAMES AND SYMPTOMS 243

INDEX BY CHINESE MEDICINALS AND FORMULAS 247

GENERAL INDEX 253

〖 Chapter 1 〗

Differentiation of Patterns and Differentiation of Diseases

Patterns are closely related to diseases. Only when one has made a clear pattern differentiation can the disease be understood and treated. Pattern differentiation and disease differentiation are inseparable. In the *Shāng Hán Lùn* (On Cold Damage, 伤寒论), the description of *guì zhī* (Ramulus Cinnamomi, 桂枝) pattern and *chái hú* (Radix Bupleuri, 柴胡) pattern include the disease location and the disease cause. For instance, in *taiyang* disease, "When *Guì Zhī Tāng* (Cinnamon Twig Decoction, 桂枝汤) has been taken, or purging has been used, and there is still stiffness and pain in the head and nape, there is low fever, no sweating, stomach fullness, slight pain, and difficult urination, *Guì Zhī Tāng* (Cinnamon Twig Decoction) minus *guì zhī* (Ramulus Cinnamomi) plus *fú líng* (Poria, 茯苓) and *bái zhú* (Rhizoma Atractylodis Macrocephalae, 白术) governs." This is an example of using treatment methods to indicate pattern differentiation without the differentiation of disease. Although the *Shāng Hán Lùn* (On Cold Damage) focuses on pattern differentiation and the *Jīn Guì Yào Lüè* (Essential Prescriptions of the Golden Coffer, 金匮要略) concentrates on disease differentiation, they supplement each other.

What does disease mean? What is a pattern? A disease manifests first and then a pattern appears. Disease is the root while pattern is the manifestation. Disease does not change but pattern varies frequently. So the study of pattern differentiation must be based on disease. For example, last year's Damp-Warmth was a yang pattern, but this year's Damp-Warmth is a yin pattern. The dysentery yesterday was feverish, but the dysentery today has counterflow cold; in the morning there is no fever, but in the afternoon a high fever begins; the patient had no appetite in the evening, but the next morning he is hungry. These examples show how changeable pattern is, even though the disease remains the same. That is why disease is easy to diagnose, but pattern is difficult to differentiate. If the pattern is correctly differentiated, the disease will be correctly and effectively treated.

In the human body, the four limbs and bones of the whole body, the five *zang* organs and the six *fu* organs all have special functions. When a single *zang* organ, a *fu* organ, a tendon, or a bone is in disorder, all the viscera will be affected and related symptoms and signs will manifest. If the disease is located in the stomach, digestive patterns will appear; if the disease is located in the lung, respiratory patterns will appear. The pattern that appears first is called the main pattern, a pattern that appears later and affects the whole body is known as a secondary pattern. Although each of them is called a pattern, they are different and should be treated differently.

Take gastritis for example. It may be characterized by stomach pain and increased appetite, or by no pain and poor appetite, or by nausea and vomiting, or by diarrhea, or by constipation, or by floating edema, or by fever, or by headache. These are various secondary patterns. Since secondary pattern are different, *Guì Zhī Rén Shēn Tāng* (Cinnamon Twig and Ginseng Decoction, 桂枝人参汤), or *Chái Hú Tāng* (Bupleurum Decoction, 柴胡汤), or *Lǐ Zhōng Tāng* (Middle Regulating Decoction, 理中汤), or *Chéng Qì Tāng* (Purgative Decoction, 承气汤), or *Xiè Xīn Tāng* (Heart Draining Decoction, 泻心汤) can be used to treat both the primary pattern and the secondary pattern. For example, the primary pattern treated by *Rén Shēn Tāng* (Ginseng Decoction, 人参汤) is characterized by epigastric focal distention and hardness and chest painful obstruction. The secondary pattern treated by it is characterized by: vomiting, diarrhea, frequent spitting, acute stomach pain, difficulty in urination, etc.

For instance, if a patient presents with epigastric focal distention and chest painful obstruction as the main pattern, and at the same time has urinary difficulty and frequent spitting, then *Rén Shēn Tāng* (Ginseng Decoction) will work well. So when a doctor chooses medicine to treat the disease, he mut be very clear about the primary pattern and the secondary pattern of the disease. If the medicine used does not agree with the pattern and if the primary pattern is confused with the secondary pattern, it will inevitably lead to a deteriorated pattern.

If the patient needs sweating but the doctor tries to prevent sweating, or if the patient needs consolidation but he is drained instead, or if the patient needs to be treated by warming therapy but the doctor uses cooling methods, or if the patient needs to be treated by cooling therapy but the doctor uses warming therapy, this is contrary to the disease conditions, and this is called counteractive treatment. Counteractive treatment results in symptoms called contrary pattern. Contrary patterns change rapidly and are difficult to cure.

Deteriorated patterns and contrary patterns are both caused by wrong treatment. The *Shāng Hán Lùn* (On Cold Damage) has recorded various therapeutic methods to deal with deteriorated and abnormal patterns. The patterns caused by improper use of medicines or incorrect methods in cultivating health are called false patterns.

A fixed pattern is called the normal pattern while a changeable pattern is called an abnormal pattern. For example, the normal pattern treated by *Rén Shēn Tāng* (Ginseng Decoction) is marked by epigastric focal distention and hardness, difficulty in urination, or acute epigastric pain and painful chest obstruction, or epigastric focal distention and qi knotted in the chest. If there are symptoms such as vomiting, headache, fever, whole-body pain, aversion to cold, and aversion to drinking, it is an abnormal pattern. So when diagnosing patterns, doctors must carefully differentiate yin and yang, internal and external, deficiency and excess, and cold and heat aspects of the disease in question. If a doctor is able to understand the primary pattern, he is certainly able to prevent and treat the secondary pattern. If a doctor understands the normal pattern, he can surely prevent abnormal patterns.

Zhang Zhong-jing (张仲景)'s suggestion of pattern differentiation by taking the pulse is an example of the idea that treatment of disease must focus on the root cause as described in the *Huáng Dì Nèi Jīng* (Yellow Emperor's Inner Canon, 黄帝内经). "Root cause" refers to either the common cause of all diseases or the specific cause of one single disease. Both aspects should be emphasized in diagnosis and treatment. Both the *Shāng Hán Lùn* (On Cold Damage) and the *Jīn Guì Yào Lüè* (Essential Prescriptions of the Golden Coffer) address the root cause of diseases, so the formulas in these texts are very effective.

In treating diseases, one uses formulas. Among patients with diseases, some are "ripe" and some are "not yet ripe". As to the ripe ones, one formula is used to treat one disease; as to the unripe ones, several formulas have to be used to treat one disease. Therefore, in the *Shāng Hán Lùn* (On Cold Damage), it says that certain formulas "govern" or "master" a disease, while others "can be used," and still others "are suitable."

Treatment based on pattern differentiation is typical of traditional Chinese medicine. This idea first appeared in the Chapter of *Zhì Zhēn Yào Dà Lùn* (Great Treatise on the Essentials of Supreme Truth, 至真要大论) in the *Nei Jing Sù Wèn* (Plain Questions, 素问), but it was Zhang Zhong-jing who further developed it and made it practical. The *Shāng Hán Lùn* (On Cold Damage) says, *"In taiyang disease for three days in which the patient has already been sweated, if it cannot be relieved by vomiting therapy, purgation therapy, or warm needling, it is a deteriorated disease. It cannot be treated by guì zhī (Ramulus Cinnamomi). One must carefully examine the pulse to make sure of the disease cause and then treat it according to the pattern."* In the Chapter on Differentiation of *shaoyang* Disease Pulse Patterns and Treatment in the *Shāng Hán Lùn* (On Cold Damage), it says, *"If taiyang disease is not relieved and is transmitted to the shaoyang, there will appear such symptoms as hypochondriac hardness and fullness, dry heaves, inability to eat, and alternating cold and heat. If it has not been treated by vomiting or purgation therapies, and the pulse is deep and tight, it can be treated by Xiǎo Chái Hú Tāng (Minor Bupleurum Decoction,*

小柴胡汤). *If the patient has already been treated by the methods of vomiting, purgation, sweating, or warm needling, and delirium appears, then this is a deteriorated pattern, and is no longer a Chái Hú Tāng (Bupleurum Decoction) pattern. One must examine the disease cause and then treat it according to the pattern.*"

Disease appears first and patterns appear later. So the study of patterns must be based on the analysis of disease. Disease is either Cold Damage (*Shāng Hán*, 伤寒), warm disease(*Wēn Bìng*, 温病), or Miscellaneous (*Zá Bìng*, 杂病). When a doctor diagnoses disease, he should first make it clear whether it is caused by internal damage or external attack. If it is external, is it Cold Damage or Warm Disease? If it is Cold Damage, care should be taken to make clear whether it is *taiyang*, *yangming*, or *shaoyang*, or whether it is *taiyin*, *shaoyin*, or *jueyin*. If it is a *taiyang* disease, it should be further analyzed to see whether it is Wind Strike or Cold Damage. Only when such careful analysis is made can one decide to use *Guì Zhī Tāng* (Cinnamon Twig Decoction), *Má Huáng Tāng* (Ephedra Decoction, 麻黄汤), or *Qīng Lóng Tāng* (Blue Green Dragon Decoction, 青龙汤). Only by doing so can a doctor be clear about how to use sweating therapy, purgation therapy, tonification therapy, and clearing therapy.

Usually there is one specific formula for one specific disease. However, sometimes one single pattern may be composed of several other patterns. For example, headache is one pattern and fever is another pattern. But how can one know when to use *Má Huáng Tāng* (Ephedra Decoction), when to use *Guì Zhī Tāng* (Cinnamon Twig Decoction), or when to use *Gě Gēn Tāng* (Pueraria Decoction, 葛根汤) to treat headache? How can one know whether the fever is caused by external attack or by miscellaneous disease? It is not easy to do. Furthermore, disease is demonstrated by patterns. For instance, the symptoms of floating pulse, fever and aversion to cold indicate Cold Damage, while the symptoms of thirst and no aversion to cold indicate Warm Disease.

Doctors in ancient times differentiated patterns in order to know the changes of disease, the advance and retreat of pathogenic factors, and the rise and fall of the healthy qi (*Zhèng qì*, 正气). For example, with Cold Damage, in the first day of attack, it affects the *taiyang*. If the pulse appears quiescent, it will not transmit. If the patient wants to vomit and appears restless and the pulse is rapid, then the disease will transmit. After six or seven days, if there is no high fever and the patient appears restless, it shows that yang has entered yin. Three days after the initial attack of Cold Damage, the disease has penetrated through the three yang channels and begins to invade the three yin channels. If the patient is able to eat without vomiting, it shows that the three yin channels have not been attacked. If *taiyang* disease is treated by purgation therapy, qi will rush up. This can be treated with *Guì Zhī Tāng* (Cinnamon Twig Decoction). If qi does not rush up, this formula should not be used. With Cold Damage, if the yang pulse is choppy and the yin pulse is wiry, there will be acute abdominal pain, which can be treated by *Xiǎo Jiàn Zhōng Tāng* (Minor Center Fortifying Decoction, 小建中汤). If this does not help, then *Xiǎo Chái Hú Tāng* (Minor Bupleurum Decoction) can be used. In the *Shāng Hán Lùn* (On Cold Damage), it is said that if the patient feels thirsty after taking *Chái Hú Tāng* (Radix Bupleuri Decoctioin), then the disease now belongs to the *yangming*, and one should use these methods to treat it. In describing *taiyang* disease, it says that if the pulse appears deep instead of floating, it indicates that the disease has entered the yin from the yang. *Shaoyin* disease does not show the symptom of fever; if there is fever, it means that the disease has changed from yin into yang.

Pattern differentiation allows the doctor to understand the causes of diseases among different people, so that the same disease may be treated with different therapies and different diseases may be treated with the same therapy. For example, diseases caused by pathogenic dampness are characterized either by edema, by diarrhea, or by difficult urination. If the diseases are different but the treatment methods used are the same, it is known as using the same therapy for different diseases. If the causes are different but the diseases are the same, then they should be treated with different therapies. If the diseases are the same but the locations are different, they should also be treated with different therapies. For example, in edema, if it is located above the waist, sweating therapy should be used; if edema is located below the waist, one should promote urination. If the causes of diseases are the same, but the locations are different and the patterns are also different, then the therapeutic methods must also be different. For example, if pathogenic dampness attacks the stomach, it will cause vomiting; if it attacks the spleen, it will cause diarrhea. If there is a combined disease of two yang channels, it will lead to diarrhea. This means the disease is in the intestines, which can be treated by *Gě Gēn Tāng* (Pueraria Decoction). If there is no diarrhea but vomiting, it shows that the disease is located in the stomach, which can be treated by *Gě Gēn Tāng* (Pueraria Decoction) plus *bàn xià* (Rhizoma Pinelliae). In treating different diseases with the same therapy, *Shèn Qì Wán* (Kidney-Qi Pill, 肾气丸) in the *Jīn Guì Yào Lüè* (Essential Prescriptions of the Golden Coffer, 金匮要略) is a good example. There are five uses of *Shèn Qì Wán* in the *Jīn Guì Yào Lüè* (Essential Prescriptions of the Golden Coffer): the first one is for treating abdominal numbness after Wind Stroke; the second one is for treating deficiency-taxation, with symptoms such as cramping pain of the lower abdomen and difficulty in urination; the third one is for treating disorders of phlegm retention and shortness of breath; the fourth one is for treating insomnia in women due to vexation heat and difficult urination; the fifth one is for treating wasting and thirsting disease.

The *Shāng Hán Lùn* (On Cold Damage) puts an emphasis on pattern differentiation in order to treat incorrect treatment, while the *Jīn Guì Yào Lüè* (Essential Prescriptions of the Golden Coffer) focuses on disease differentiation, using a specific formula for a specific disease. For example, in the *Jīn Guì*, in the chapter talking about *Bǎi Hé* (lily disease) and *Hú Huò* (erosion of the mouth, eye, and genitalia, or Behcet's disease), it says that "*A patient with Bǎi Hé (lily disease) disease wants to eat but cannot, is often silent, wants to sleep but cannot, wants to move but cannot, has a bitter taste in the mouth and red urine. No medicines can help because, when taking medicines, the patient will immediately suffer from acute vomiting and diarrhea.*" The patterns in this disease often fluctuate. That is why it says no medicines can help. But when treated by *bǎi hé* (Bulbus Lilii), all the symptoms are relieved. Take *Hú Huò* (erosion of the mouth, eye, and genitalia, 狐惑) for another example. It appears like Cold Damage disease, characterized by sleepiness, erosion of the mouth and the genitalia. *Yī Zōng Jīn Jiàn* (Golden Mirror of Medicine, 医宗金鉴) regards it as syphilis. Doctors in different dynasties understood it differently. Although it involves the throat and anus, it does not pertain to throat patterns, rectal patterns or gynecological patterns. In the *Jīn Guì Yào Lüè* (Essential Prescriptions of the Golden Coffer), *Gān Cǎo Xiè Xīn Tāng* (Licorice heart Draining Decoction, 甘草泻心汤) is used to treat both *Hú Huò* (erosion of the mouth, eye, and genitalia) and gastric ulcer. This is a good example of treating different diseases with the same therapy.

Malaria, marked by chills followed by fever, is another example. There appear the symptoms of vexation, thirst, and severe headache. After profuse sweating, it will be alleviated. It often attacks regularly. When it does not attack, the patient appears normal. One should first differentiate this disease and then using sweating therapy.

A patient named Han suffered from lower abdominal pain. He went to several provinces to look for treatment. After many years his illness was not cured. When he came to see me, I found that his problem matched the description in the *Jīn Guì Yào Lüè* (Essential Prescriptions of the Golden Coffer) about Cold Hernia. So I prescribed *Wū Tóu Guì Zhī Tāng* (Radix Aconiti and Ramulus Cinnamomi Decoction, 乌头桂枝汤) and his illness was cured.

In modern times, diseases like rheumatic arthritis are often regarded as incurable. However, for years I have used *Guì Zhī Sháo Yào Zhī Mǔ Tāng* (Cinnamon Twig, Peony and Rhizoma Anemarrhenae Decoction, 桂枝芍药知母汤) to cure many people with arthritis. Another example is Meniere's syndrome, known as dizziness in ancient times, which is actually caused by invasion of water and can be effectively treated by *Líng Guì Zhú Gān Tāng* (Poria, Cinnamon Twig, Atractylodes Macrocephala and Licorice Decoction, 苓桂术甘汤) and *Xiǎo Bàn Xià Tāng* (Minor Pinellia Decoction, 小半夏汤) plus *lóng gǔ* (Os Draconis), *mǔ lì* (Concha Ostreae), *chén pí* (Pericarpium Citri Reticulatae), *fú líng* (Poria), and *zé xiè* (Rhizoma Alismatis). Another example is the use of *guā lóu* (Fructus Trichosanthis) and *xiè bái* (Bulbus Allii Macrostami) to treat Painful Chest Obstruction. Also, *Chái Hú Lóng Gǔ Mǔ Lì Tāng* (Radix Bupleuri, Os Draconis and Ostrea Decoction, 柴胡龙骨牡蛎汤) can be used to treat epilepsy; *Qiān Jīn Wěi Jìng Tāng* (Phragmites Stem Decoction, 千金苇茎汤) can be used to treat respiratory tract infection in bronchiectasis; pills of *shè xiāng* (Moschus), developed by Xu Shu-wei (许叔微), can be used to treat sciatica; *Xiǎo Jiàn Zhōng Tāng* (Minor Center Fortifying Decoction) can be used to treat gastroptosis.

Some doctors, like Xue Li-zhai (薛立斋), Zhao Yang-kui (赵养葵) and Cheng Zhong-ling (程钟龄), only concentrated on the root cause of all diseases, but not on the root cause of individual diseases. However, the *Jīn Guì Yào Lüè* (Essential Prescriptions of the Golden Coffer) and the *Shāng Hán Lùn* (On Cold Damage) concentrate on both the common cause of all diseases and the specific cause of individual diseases. Take Wind-Warmth disease and Damp-Warmth disease for example. Wind and Damp are the specific causes while Warmth is a common cause to both. Treatment based on pattern differentiation means to differentiate the disease first and then differentiate the patterns. A disease with headache is a pattern and a disease with foot pain is another. So the treatment should focus on the head and the foot respectively. At the same time, cautions should be taken to deal with combined patterns.

There are specific formulas for specific disease, but patients are different in constitution, age, and duration of the disease, so a disease will manifest differently in each person. For instance, the disease treated by *Xiǎo Chái Hú Tāng* (Minor Bupleurum Decoction) is marked by vexation without vomiting, or thirst, or abdominal pain, or focal distention and hardness below the ribs, or epigastric palpitations and difficult urination, or no thirst but low fever, or cough, and other various different symptoms. Although these symptoms will never appear in one single patient, the main patterns to be treated by *chái hú* (Radix Bupleuri) remain unchanged. Within different patterns, there must be one that is the main pattern. For *chái hú* (Radix Bupleuri), the main pattern is composed of three different aspects: alternating cold and heat; bitter taste in the mouth, dry throat and dizziness; discomfort and fullness in the chest and hypochondria, and dry heaves. However, discomfort and fullness in the chest and hypochondria is the principal aspect within the main pattern. In order to understand the source of disease and be adaptable in one's treatments, then one must use treatments based on pattern differentiation.

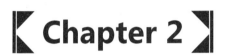

Chapter 2

Pathogenesis and Treatment of Coronary Heart Disease

Coronary atherosclerosis is a disease in modern medicine. This disease does not exist in traditional Chinese medicine. However, its clinical manifestations, such as Painful Chest Obstruction, chest oppression, palpitations, and shortness of breath, can be found in classical traditional Chinese medical books like the *Sù Wèn* (Plain Questions) and the *Líng Shū* (Spiritual Pivot, 灵枢) in the *Huáng Dì Nèi Jīng* (Yellow Emperor's Inner Canon). Zhang Zhong-jing also described a disease in the *Jīn Guì Yào Lüè* (Essential Prescriptions of the Golden Coffer) marked by Painful Chest-Obstruction, insomnia, and heart pain that extends through to the back. These books provide practical and effective therapeutic methods. In reality, the description of the so-called Painful Chest Obstruction (Xiōng Bì, 胸痹) in traditional Chinese medicine is quite similar to the manifestations of coronary heart disease.

Understanding Coronary Heart Disease in Chinese Medicine

According to Chinese medicine theory, Painful Chest Obstruction and heart pain are related to the heart, the lung, the blood vessels and the stomach. The intake of nutrients, discharge of waste, and the activities of sweating and respiration all depend on blood circulation. The blood, however, relies on heart-yang to propel its normal circulation. Thus it is said that, *"the heart is the root of life, and its abundance is in the blood vessels."* The heart, the great yang within yang, is located in the chest. If yang in the upper *jiao* is deficient, it means the heart-yang is slightly weak. If the heart-yang is weak, it will affect blood flow and cause blood stagnation, which eventually leads to chest pain. As blood stasis and turbid yin builds, then eventually this can lead to myocardial infarction. That is why it is believed this disease is related to the cardiac and pulmonary vessels.

In the Chapter on Painful Chest-Obstruction and Shortness of Breath in the *Jīn Guì Yào Lüè* (Essential Prescriptions of the Golden Coffer), it says that a weak yang pulse and a wiry yin pulse indicate Painful Chest-Obstruction. The root cause of this problem is extreme deficiency. The weak yang in the upper *jiao* is shown in the weak yang pulse. This weak yang leads to blood deficiency, which in turn is shown in the wiry yin pulse.

In the Chapter on Vomiting, Nausea and Diarrhea in the *Jīn Guì Yào Lüè* (Essential Prescriptions of the Golden Coffer), there is this dialogue:

"The student asked: The pulse of the patient is rapid and a rapid pulse indicates heat. So the treatment should focus on promoting digestion, yet instead vomiting therapy is used. Why?

The master answered: Inducing sweating weakens the yang and the diaphragm qi. A rapid pulse shows that there is pathogenic heat inside the body. Thus one cannot promote digestion, because there is cold in the stomach. Wiry pulse is deficiency. If the stomach qi is deficient, one who eats in the morning will vomit in the evening. This is stomach regurgitation."

In the same chapter it also says that a weak and rapid pulse indicates deficient qi. If qi is deficient, blood will become deficient. If blood is deficient, there will be cold inside the chest. Qi deficiency in the diaphragm means deficiency of heart yang; deficiency-cold inside the stomach means decline of stomach yang. Excessive sweating will make yang weak and deficiency of qi in the diaphragm will make stomach qi insufficient and unable to digest food. Nutritive qi (*yíng qì*, 营气), defensive qi (*wèi qì*, 卫气) and chest qi (*zōng qì*, 宗气) all come from the middle *jiao*. If food cannot be digested, these three kinds of qi will gradually weaken, eventually leading to insufficiency of qi inside the chest.

In the Chapter on Painful Obstruction in the *Sù Wèn* (Plain Questions), it says that Painful Obstruction of the heart means obstruction of the vessels. If the vessels are obstructed, heart qi will certainly become deficient, leading to coldness in the chest and decline of stomach yang, which weakens digestion. This is what causes vomiting and diarrhea. The production of nutritive qi, defensive qi, and chest qi all depend on stomach yang, since it is responsible for digesting food. If yang in the chest is weak, it will affect blood circulation and cause Painful Chest Obstruction. Both the classics and clinical experience show that coronary heart disease is caused by a decline of yang in the chest, heart blood deficiency, and abnormalities of blood circulation. Therefore, coronary heart disease is a sort of excess disease caused by deficiency; deficiency is the root aspect and excess is secondary. The heart, the blood vessels, and the stomach are all related. The stomach receives food and governs digestion; the spleen governs transportation and moves stomach fluids, bringing nutrients from food to the entire body. As to the nutritive qi, defensive qi and chest qi, the chest qi accumulates inside the chest, the nutritive qi flows inside the vessels, and the defensive qi flows outside the vessels. The vessels are considered an extraordinary *fu* organ, and are governed by the heart. The heart is characterized by beating. Usually it beats four times within each breath. The *Sù Wèn* (Plain Questions) says that the major collateral of the stomach is called "*xū lǐ* (虚里)," which penetrates through the diaphragm and is connected with the lung, emerges below the left breast and causes a beating movement that can be seen through the clothes. This area below the left breast is where the apex of the heart is located. This place is called the major collateral of the stomach and is also known as the chest qi. According to modern medicine, severe angina pectoris is often accompanied by nausea, vomiting, and distention in the upper abdomen. Excessive intake of rich food can also cause angina pectoris. This shows that traditional Chinese medicine is correct when it says that the heart is related to the stomach.

Causes of Coronary Heart Disease

• Excessive intake of rich food:

The *Sù Wèn* (Plain Questions) says that food taken into the stomach is not yet separated into turbid and essence aspects. This turbid essence flows into the vessels, which home to the heart. Excessive intake of rich foods can block the major collateral of the stomach, which obstructs the flow of blood, depriving the heart of its nourishment, resulting in pain.

• Psychological factors:

The *Sù Wèn* (Plain Questions) says that if yang qi is refined, the spirit will be cultivated, and if the yang qi is soft, the sinews will be nourished; if the yin qi is quiet, the spirit will be stored, and if it is rash and impetuous, one will wither away. The *Líng Shū* (Divine Pivot) says that the various emotions can damage the spirit and weaken the body. Clinical experience shows that coronary heart disease is often caused by psychological factors.

• Climatic factors:

According to the *Sù Wèn* (Plain Questions), invasion of Cold into the vessels will prevent blood from flowing and cause sudden pain.

This disease is caused by sudden blockage of the vessels due to cold invasion, which is possible because of an insufficiency of yang in the chest.

Treatment of Coronary Heart Disease

Diseases are different one from another; however they also share something in common. So for each disease, there is a special therapeutic method. For instance, in the *Jīn Guì Yào Lüè* (Essential Prescriptions of the Golden Coffer), cough marked by occasional vomiting and insomnia can be treated by *Zào Jiǎ Wán* (Fructus Gleditsiae Pill). In ancient times, the classification of diseases was strict. Take cough for example: the treatment of cough due to lung Abscess is different from that of cough due to phlegm. In order to indicate the difference in therapeutic methods, Zhang Zhong-jing discussed phlegm and Water-qi separately, and treated heart pain caused by Painful Chest Obstruction and not caused by Painful Chest Obstruction differently. Each disease has its own definite cause and therapeutic method, while patterns are different from disease because patterns show something in common. So disease does not change but patterns tend to change. For example, *Xiǎo Qīng Lóng Tāng* (Minor Blue Green Dragon Decoction, 小青龙汤) and *Xiǎo Chái Hú Tāng* (Minor Bupleurum Decoction) have their own special way of application to disease, but since patterns change, the formulas can be modified.

As to the treatment of coronary heart disease, one should make clear whether it is related to the organs, especially to the stomach. Only by doing so can one be clear about its nature and the suitable methods to be used.

● Activating Yang and removing blockage

In the *Líng Shū* (Spiritual Pivot), it says that the patient with heart disease should eat wheat, mutton, apricot and Chinese onion. It also says that acridness enters the stomach and its qi flows to the upper jiao. The upper jiao receives qi and transports it to various yang channels. In the *Explanation of the Shāng Hán Lùn (On Cold Damage)* compiled by Wang Pu-zhuang (王朴庄) in the Qing Dynasty, it says that *guā lóu* (Fructus Trichosanthis) taken by healthy people may cause interior leakage of heart-qi. Now we can use this herb to remove stagnation and invigorate yang. Yu Jia-yan (喻嘉言) said: "Painful Chest-Obstruction is caused by the flow of yin qi to the upper body due to weakness of yang qi. If the disease was mild, Zhang Zhong-jing would use alcohol with *xiè bái* (Bulbus Allii Macrostami) in order to invigorate yang; if it was severe, he would use *fù zǐ* (Radix Aconiti Lateralis Preparata) and *gān jiāng* (Rhizoma Zingiberis) to reduce yin. Ordinary doctors do not know the nature of Painful Chest-Obstruction; they often use *bái dòu kòu* (Fructus Amomi Rotundus), *guǎng mù xiāng* (Radix Aucklandiae), *hē zǐ* (Fructus Chebulae), and *sān léng* (Rhizoma Sparganii) to treat it. In fact, this method of treatment exhausts yang in the chest.

The experience of doctors in different dynasties and in our clinical practice shows that, if yang is not invigorated, blockage of the blood will occur. Also, blockage of the blood may lead to inactivation of yang. That is why clinically, heart pain due to Painful Chest-Obstruction is treated by invigorating yang to remove blockage. The formula used is *Guā Lóu Xiè Bái Bàn Xià Tāng* (Trichosanthes, Chinese Chive and Pinellia Decoction, 瓜蒌薤白半夏汤). *Guā lóu* (Fructus Trichosanthis) is used to open the chest and remove blockage in order to invigorate yang; *xiè bái* (Bulbus Allii Macrostami) is used for invigorating yang to remove blockage. Since Painful Chest-Obstruction is often marked by an upward counterflow of turbid qi of the stomach, *bàn xià* (Rhizoma Pinelliae) is used for regulating the stomach to suppress this counterflow and support heart-yang. If there is insomnia, *Suān Zǎo Rén Tāng* (Sour Jujube Decoction, 酸枣仁汤) can be used. If there is distention and fullness of the chest and lateral costal region and cold limbs, *Zhǐ Shí Xiè Bái Guì Zhī Tāng* (Immature Bitter Orange, Chinese Chive and Cinnamon Twig Decoction, 枳实薤白桂枝汤) can be used. If there is yang deficiency symptoms and sharp pain in the back, *Wū Tóu Chì Shí Zhī Wán* (Radix Aconiti and Halloysitum Rubrum Pill, 乌头赤石脂丸) can be added to the formula. If it is complicated by Visceral Agitation and Lily Disease, *Bǎi Hé Zhī Mǔ Tāng* (Bulbus Lilii and Rhizoma Anemarrhenae Decoction, 百合知母汤), *Bǎi Hé Dì Huáng Tāng* (Bulbus Lilii and Radix Rehmanniae Decoction, 百合地黄汤), *Bàn Xià Hòu Pò Tāng* (Pinellia and Officinal Magnolia Bark Decoction, 半夏厚朴汤) and *Gān Mài Dà Zǎo Tāng* (Licorice, Wheat and Jujube Decoction, 甘麦大枣汤) can be used. If the patient frequently catches cold with the symptoms of body ache and weakness, the principal formula can be used together with *Xīn Jiā Tāng* (New Additions Decoction, 新加汤).

● Combined Treatment of the heart and stomach

The heart and the stomach are closely related to each other. The stomach is the Sea of Water and Grain. Heat in the body is produced in the stomach, accumulates in the vessels and is attached to the blood. When propelled by heart-yang, it flows to all parts of the body. That is why it is said that the existence of stomach-qi indicates life while loss of stomach-qi means death. Thus the heart and the stomach depend on each other and influence each other. That is why they are treated simultaneously.

Painful Chest-Obstruction marked by blockage of qi in the chest and shortness of breath is an excess pattern that can be treated by *Jú Zhǐ Jiāng Tāng* (Fructus Citri Reticulatae, Fructus Aurantii Immaturus, and Ginger Decoction, 橘枳姜汤) with modifications. If it is marked by blockage of qi in the chest, shortness of breath, and palpitations on exertion as well as lung problems without any symptoms related to the stomach and the intestines, *Fú Líng Xìng Rén Gān Cǎo Tāng* (Poria, Semen Armeniacae Amarum and Radix Glycyrrhizae Decoction, 茯苓杏仁甘草汤) should be used. Painful Chest-Obstruction marked by stagnation of qi in the heart, retention of qi in the chest and fullness in the chest and lateral costal region is a deficiency pattern that can be treated by *Rén Shēn Tāng* (Ginseng Decoction) with the addition of other ingredients. Painful Chest-Obstruction marked by abdominal distension and fullness after meals is a deficiency pattern that can be treated by *Hòu Jiāng Bàn Gān Shēn Tāng* (Officinal Magnolia Bark, Ginger, Rhizoma Pinelliae, Licorice, and Ginseng Decoction, 厚姜半甘参汤) with modification. If there are symptoms of diarrhea and vomiting, it can be treated by *Wú Zhū Yú Tāng* (Evodia Decoction, 吴茱萸汤).

● Supplementing qi and nourishing blood

Qi and blood come from the same source but bear different names. Blood is yin while qi is yang. If there is no qi, the blood will become deficient and there will be cold in the chest. The blood is the body of qi and the qi is the function of blood. Therefore, it is said that the qi is the commander of the blood and the blood is the mother of the qi. Supplementing qi can promote blood production and nourishing the blood can invigorate qi. For example, Painful Chest-Obstruction marked by fever, no thirst, weak pulse, and deficiency of healthy qi (*Zhèng qì*), due to prolonged heart disease can be treated by *Dāng Guī Bǔ Xuè Tāng* (Chinese Angelica blood Supplementing Decoction, 当归补血汤) with the addition of other ingredients. If there is an intermittent pulse, shortness of breath, rapid pulse, and palpitations, *Dāng Guī Sháo Yào Sǎn* (Chinese Angelica and Peony Powder, 当归芍药散) can be added to the principal formula. If there are palpitations and a rapid pulse, *Shēng Mài Sǎn* (Pulse Engendering Powder, 生脉散) can be used with the addition of *suān zǎo rén* (Semen Jujubae), *lóng gǔ* (Os Draconis), *mŭ lì* (Concha Ostreae), and *dāng guī* (Radix Angelicae Sinensis). If it is marked by knotted and intermittent pulse and palpitations, *Zhì Gān Cǎo Tāng* (Honey-Fried Licorice Decoction, 炙甘草汤) can be used.

● Supporting Yang and suppressing Yin

An excess of yang causes heat and an excess of yin causes cold. Yang deficiency leads to cold while yin deficiency leads to heat. So supporting yang can suppress yin and inhibiting yin can promote yang. Painful Chest-Obstruction is caused by weakness of heart-yang, so it can be treated by supporting yang and suppressing yin. If Painful Chest-Obstruction is sometimes mild and sometimes severe, it can be treated by *Yì Yǐ Fù Zǐ Sǎn* (Coix Seed and Aconite Powder, 薏苡附子散). *Fù zǐ* (Radix Aconiti Lateralis Preparata) is used for supporting yang and *yì yǐ rén* (Semen Coicis) is used for moderating severity. If it is marked by coldness of the four limbs, indistinct pulse, and diarrhea, *Sì Nì Tāng* (Frigid Extremities Decoction, 四逆汤) can be used. If it is marked by yang deficiency and cold in the stomach, *fù zǐ* (Radix Aconiti Lateralis Preparata) can be added to the principal formula. If it is marked by stomach fullness, *Lǐ Zhōng Tāng* (Middle Regulating Decoction) is added to the principal formula. If it is marked by severe cold, *xì xīn* (Herba Asari) and *guì zhī* (Ramulus Cinnamomi) should be added to the formula.

● Activating the blood to promote flow of water

Floating edema in coronary heart disease is caused by stagnation of blood, which dilates the collaterals and causes body fluids to flow out of the vessels. In order to treat this, one should remove stagnation and activate the flow of blood. This method can be used together with methods for inducing sweating, opening the orifices, and promoting urination. Although these methods can reduce edema; they cannot prevent reoccurrence of it. The sole cause of this problem is deficiency of heart-yang. Inducing sweating, opening the orifices, and promoting urination can only reduce the edema, but cannot strengthen heart yang. An excess of water leads to a decline of yang while an excess of yang results in a decline of water. Although sweating therapy can eliminate edema, it also can disperse body heat. So for those with insufficient yang, sweating therapy may further damage yang. This is why it is said that profuse sweating causes loss of yang. Body heat is produced in the stomach and is stored in the blood. To treat those with hemorrhage, sweating therapy cannot be used; to treat those with profuse sweating, blood-letting therapy cannot be used. Thus if sweating therapy is excessively used to treat someone with yin deficiency, it will lead to a loss of body fluid. So to treat edema in coronary heart disease, *Zhēn Wǔ Tāng* (True Warrior Decoction, 真武 汤) is used to support heart yang. Other therapeutic methods can be used according to pattern differentiation to reduce edema without injuring yang. For treating floating edema due to blood stagnation, add *Dāng Guī Sháo Yào Sǎn* (Chinese Angelica and Peony Powder); for blood stasis in the lung and liver congestion, add *Shēn Sū Yǐn* (Ginseng and Perllia Beverage, 参苏饮); For edema with knotted and intermittent pulse, *Guā Lóu Xiè Bái Bàn Xià Tāng* (Trichosanthes, Chinese Chive and Pinellia Decoction) and *Zhēn Wǔ Tāng* (True Warrior Decoction) can be used together with the addition of substances that activate the blood.

● Nourishing the kidney and strengthening the tendons

The heart and the kidney mutually reinforce one another. If the kidney fails to transfer essence to the heart, the function of the heart will be weak; if the kidney fails to transfer essence to the liver, it cannot soften the liver and nourish the tendons, leading to dryness of the tendons and hardness of the vessels. This is why supplementing the kidney and nourishing the tendons is a major method used to treat Painful Chest-Obstruction. If the disease is marked by weak pulse in the Cubit (proximal) position, a slow pulse, chest oppression, palpitations, dizziness, tinnitus, low back ache, weakness of the legs, dark complexion, mild anxiety, insomnia, or hypertension, it can be treated by using *guā lóu* (Fructus Trichosanthis) and *xiè bái* (Bulbus Allii Macrostami) as the main prescription, with the addition of *Qǐ Jú Dì Huáng Wán* (Lycium Berry, Chrysanthemum and Rehmannia Pill, 杞菊地黄丸). If there is dry stool, add *cǎo jué míng* (Semen Cassiae); if there is a decline of kidney-yang with aversion to cold, cold limbs and a faint pulse, it can be treated by adding *Guì Fù Bā Wèi Wán* (Cassia Bark and Aconite Eight Ingredient Pill, 桂附八味丸) to the principal formula, or by adding *lù jiǎo jiāo* (Colla Cornus Cervi), *bā jǐ tiān* (Radix Morindae Officinalis), *xiān máo* (Rhizoma Curculiginis), *yín yáng huò* (Herba Epimedii), *dǎng shēn* (Radix Codonopsis), and *mài dōng* (Radix Ophiopogonis), or *Zuǒ Guī Wán* (Left-Restoring Pill, 左归丸) to the principal formula. If there is a knotted and intermittent pulse and palpitations, (or atrial fibrillation), *Zhì Gān Cǎo Tāng* (Honey-Fried Licorice Decoction) can be added. If there is dry stool, *huǒ má rén* (Semen Cannabis, 火麻仁) should be added; If there is insomnia, *suān zǎo rén* (Semen Ziziphi Spinosae) should be added. If there is dizziness, a wiry pulse, yin deficiency with yang floating, and hypertension, *Tiān Má Gōu Téng Yǐn* (Gastrodia and Uncaria Beverage, 天麻钩藤饮) or *Qǐ Jú Dì Huáng Wán* (Lycium Berry, Chrysanthemum and Rehmannia Pill) can be used in addition to the primary formula.

Conclusion

1. Painful Chest-Obstruction is comprised of heart pain and pertains to coronary heart disease in modern medicine. According to Chinese medicine, it is a disease located in the heart but closely related to the spleen, stomach, kidney, liver, and lung.

2. This disease is a deficiency pattern caused by deficiency of heart and stomach yang, decline of kidney yang, yin deficiency in the liver and kidney as well as failure of the lung qi to disperse.

3. This disease is caused by weakness of the healthy qi and injury of the viscera, not by invasion of exogenous pathogenic factors. It should be diagnosed and treated by differentiation of both the disease and the pattern.

4. Cold in the chest in Painful Chest-Obstruction is due to yang deficiency. Attack of exterior cold does not cause this condition, but it can trigger it. That is why it can be cured without warm dispersing herbs. Clinical practice shows that the main treatment method should be dipersing yang and opening the Painful Obstruction, while at the same time supporting yang, invigorating the blood and moving qi. If one does not focus on weakness of yang and healthy qi deficiency as the root of this disease, then, even though he may get an immediate effect, over the course of time it will be difficult to avoid consuming the patient's yang and damaging his yin.

〖 Chapter 3 〗

Treatment of Chronic Cardiopulmonary Disease

From 1962-1963, I have treated eight cases of chronic pneumocardial disease with a significant curative effect. Among the eight patients, two were hospitalized twice. They suffered from severe heart failure when they entered the hospital. They were mainly treated with Chinese herbs. Western medicine was used occasionally if necessary. For example, digitalis was used to treat two of the patients and a small dosage of diuretics was used to treat five of the patients. Sometimes antibiotics and aminophylline were also used.

Chinese Medicine Diagnosis

● Observation:

Listless spirit, shortness of breath with rapid breath, pale complexion, swollen eyelids, cyanotic lips, and bluish nails; cyanotic tongue in two cases; blackish tongue in four cases; normal tongue in two cases; thin white greasy tongue coating in five cases; and grayish tongue coating in one case.

● Listening/smelling:

Hoarse voice and rapid breath are in eight cases; frequent cough are in six cases; intermittent cough are in two cases; gurgling noise are in the throat in two cases.

● Asking:

Included history of chronic cough with excessive phlegm and liability to cold attack; excessive sticky phlegm in six cases; shortness of breath, chest oppression, epigastric focal distention, abdominal distension, scanty inhibited urination and gradual-onset edema in all patients; palpitations in seven patients; and frequent sweating in two patients.

● **Touching:**

Edema of varied degrees (can reach pitting edema) and cold extremities in all eight cases; ascites in three cases; slippery pulse in four cases; thin and rapid pulse in four cases.

Treatment Based on Pattern Differentiation

Chronic pulmonary heart disease pertains to retention of phlegm and fluids, cough and dyspnea and Water qi in Chinese medicine. The root cause is yang deficiency of the heart and the kidney; the branch cause is retention of phlegm and fluids and lung obstruction. If the disease is marked by stagnation of lung qi, severe panting and cough, excessive phlegm, aversion to cold and fever, it can be treated by *Xiǎo Qīng Lóng Tāng* (Minor Blue Green Dragon Decoction) first to scatter cold and remove pathogenic factors. If there is internal heat, *shí gāo* (Gypsum Fibrosum) can be added. If the superficial pattern is mild and heart and kidney yang is deficient, the treatment should focus on warming yang to diffuse the lung and draining water. *Zhēn Wǔ Tāng* (True Warrior Decoction) combined with *Yuè Bì Tāng* (Maidservant From Yue Decoction, 越婢汤), with modifications, should be used. If the edema is severe, one should unblock yang and drain water. The formula used is *Xiāo Shuǐ Shèng Yù Tāng* (Reduce Water to Sagely Cure Decoction, 消水圣愈汤). This is actually *Guì Zhī Tāng* (Cinnamon Twig Decoction) with the deletion of *sháo yào* (Chinese herbaceoous peony) and the addition of *má huáng* (Herba Ephedrae), *fù zǐ* (Radix Aconiti Lateralis Preparata), *xì xīn* (Herba Asari), and *zhī mǔ* (Rhizoma Anemarrhenae). If heart and kidney yang are deficient and concurrently the heart and lung qi and yin are insufficient, one should warm yang and transform water, tonify qi, and generate fluids. The formula used is *Zhēn Wǔ Tāng* (True Warrior Decoction) combined with *Shēng Mài Sǎn* (Pulse Engendering Powder) with the addition of herbs for resolving phlegm and eliminating dampness. If the edema is severe, herbs for draining water can be added, such as *chē qián zǐ* (Semen Plantaginis) 30g and *bái máo gēn* (Rhizoma Imperatae) 30g; or herbs for invigorating the blood can be added, such as *sū mù* (Lignum Sappan), *táo rén* (Semen Persicae) and *ǒu jié* (Nodus Nelumbinis). If there are only the symptoms of cough with phlegm, shortness of breath, and chest stuffiness, it means that heart yang is begining to decline, phlegm-damp is stagnating, and lung qi is not diffusing properly. This can be treated by regulating the lung and the stomach. One should use *Wēn Dǎn Tāng* (Gallbladder Warming Decoction, 温胆汤) with the addition of *xìng rén* (Semen Armeniacae Amarum), *jié gěng* (Radix Platycodi), *chuān bèi mǔ* (Bulbus Fritillariae Cirrhosae), *yì yǐ rén* (Semen Coicis), *zǐ wǎn* (Radix Asteris, 紫菀), and *shēng jiāng* (Rhizoma Zingiberis Recens). If there is prolonged cough with yin deficiency and lung heat, use herbs that clear the lung, transform phlegm, and nourish yin, such as *zhú rú* (Caulis Bambusae in Taeniam), *shā shēn* (Radix Adenophorae Strictae), *mài dōng* (Radix Ophiopogonis), *huáng qín* (Radix Scutellariae), and *guā lóu* (Fructus Trichosanthis). In order to nourish the heart, one can use *fú xiǎo mài* (Fructus Tritici Levis), *yuǎn zhì* (Radix Polygalae) and *guì zhī* (Ramulus Cinnamomi). If there is panting and a gurgling noise in the throat, *Shè Gān Má Huáng Tāng* (Belamcanda and Ephedra Decoction, 射干麻黄汤) can be used.

Clinical Treatment

Heart failure in all eight cases was controlled within two weeks and no patient died. In all cases, the edema disappeared, the liver returned to normal, dyspnea was alleviated, and the palpitations, shortness of breath, cough, and chest oppression were improved.

【 Case Study 】

Patient Deng, a housewife from Hebei Province, 48 years old, married. On June 15, 1963 she came to the hospital. She had suffered with edema and shortness of breath for half a year, which had worsened within the last week. She caught a cold in January 1961 and began to suffer from cough, shortness of breath, and lower limb edema, which were improved after treatment, but she frequently had palpitations, especially in the last month. The clinical manifestations were palpitations immediately after movement, shortness of breath, lower limb edema, epigastric focal distention, cough, vomiting of white phlegm, and scanty urine. Physical examination revealed a wiry, thin, and rapid pulse, white tongue coat, rapid breath, slight edema of the face, cyanotic lips, and distention of the jugular veins.

[Pattern differentiation]

Yang deficiency of the heart and kidney, retention of water and fluids inside, blockage of phlegm and dampness, and stagnation of lung qi. The treatment should focus on clearing and diffusing the lung, descending qi, transforming phlegm, and warming yang. The formula used was *Yuè Bì Tāng* (Maidservant From Yue Decoction) combined with *Zhēn Wǔ Tāng* (True Warrior Decoction), with modifications.

[Formula]

Chinese Name	Pin Yin	Amount	Latin Name
生石膏	*shēng shí gāo*	12g	Gypsum Fbrosum
麻黄	*má huáng*	3g	Herba Ephedrae
甘草	*gān cǎo*	9g	Radix Glycyrrhizae
云苓	*yún líng*	12g	Poria from Yunnan Province of China
白术	*bái zhú*	9g	Rhizoma Atractylodis Macrocephalae
白芍	*bái sháo*	9g	Raidix Paeoniae Alba
附子	*fù zǐ*	6g	Radix Aconiti Lateralis Preparata
生姜	*shēng jiāng*	9g	Rhizoma Zingiberis Recens
大枣	*dà zǎo*	5g	Fructus Jujubae
车前子	*chē qián zǐ*	15g	Semen Plantaginis
白茅根	*bái máo gēn*	30g	Rhizoma Imperatae
杏仁	*xìng rén*	9g	Semen Armeniacae Amarum

[Results]

After taking three doses of the formula, her urination was increased to 1500-1900ml each day and the lower limbs edema was markedly improved. After five doses of the formula, the edema disappeared, the liver returned to normal, and the cough was alleviated. Then the formula was modified with the addition of *hòu pò* (Cortex Magnoliae Officinalis) 6g and *chén pí* (Pericarpium Citri Reticulatae) 6g. After treatment, her panting was reduced, but the chest oppression remained unchanged. So *bái máo gēn* (Rhizoma Imperatae), *chē qián zǐ* (Semen Plantaginis) and *hòu pò* (Cortex Magnoliae Officinalis) were deleted from the formula, and 9g of *sū zǐ* (Fructus Perillae, 苏子) was added. After taking five more doses, her symptoms improved, but she still had a cough. Therefore, the treatment methods of expanding the chest, regulating the qi, and clearing the lung were used. The formula was *Hòu Pò Má Huáng Tāng* (Official Magnolia Bark and Ephedra Decoction, 厚朴麻黄汤) with modification.

[Formula]

Chinese Name	Pin Yin	Amount	Latin Name
厚朴	hòu pò	6g	Cortex Magnoliae Officinalis
麻黄	má huáng	3g	Herba Ephedrae
半夏	bàn xià	9g	Rhizoma Pinelliae
杏仁	xìng rén	9g	Semen Armeniacae Amarum
甘草	gān cǎo	9g	Radix Glycyrrhizae
沙参	shā shēn	18g	Radix Adenophorae Strictae
小麦	xiǎo mài	30g	Fructus Tritici
茯苓	fú líng	9g	Poria
细辛	xì xīn	3g	Herba Asari
五味子	wǔ wèi zǐ	6g	Fructus Schizandrae
生姜	shēng jiāng	4.5g	Rhizoma Zingiberis Recens

After taking this formula, all symptoms were significantly improved and the condition of the patient was stabilized.

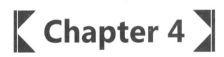

Chapter 4

Treatment of Myocarditis

Clinical practice shows that myocarditis is a complication of warm disease because exterior pathogenic factors in warm diseasemay attack the heart muscles at a late stage of the disease.

Chinese medicine holds that the heart is connected with the vessels and the vessels are the pathways of the blood. The nutrient qi flows inside and the defensive qi flows outside of the vessels. Both the nutrient qi and defensive qi come from the middle *jiao* and converge in the heart and the lung. When pathogenic factors attack the body, they first attack the nutrient qi and defensive qi. After invasion of the body, pathogenic factors may enter the heart through the vessels and cause shortness of breath, mental fatigue, tidal fever, rapid, intermittent, and knotted pulse. Wrong treatment may damage yin and yang, eventually leading to an indistinct pulse, cold limbs, pale tongue, and low-grade fever. In the clinic, one also sees Warm Toxin pathogens burning the interior, directly damaging the nutrient qi and blood, entering the heart, and causing such symptoms as rapid and weak pulse, fever and palpitations, red tongue, and shortness of breath.This pattern is caused by invasion of the heart by Warm Toxin. Therefore, the treatment should focus on removing toxin and clearing blood-heat. One should be careful to see if either the yin or the yang has been damaged. At the early stage, the treatment method should be to remove the toxin, nourish yin, and clear heat. The formula used is *Zhú Yè Shí Gāo Tāng* (Lophatherum and Gypsum Decoction, 竹叶石膏汤) with the addition of other ingredients, such as *gé gēn* (Radix Puerariae) 18g; *lián qiào* (Fructus Forsythiae) 15g; *shēng dì* (Radix Rehmanniae) 30g; *zǐ huā dì dīng* (Herba Violae) 12g; *pú gōng yīng* (Herba Taraxaci) 30g; and *jīn yín huā* (Flos Lonicerae) 15g. In order to nourish yin and clear heat, the formula used is *Shēng Mài Sǎn* (Pulse Engendering Powder) combined with *Yī Guàn Jiān* (Effective Integration Decoction, 一贯煎), with the addition of *zhī zǐ* (Fructus Gardeniae, 栀子), *dān pí* (Cortex Moutan Radicis), *chuān huáng lián* (Rhizoma Coptidis from Sichuan Province of China), and *pú gōng yīng* (Herba

Taraxaci). Treatment at the early stage mainly focuses on the blood level.

The method used at the middle stage focuses on supporting healthy qi and eliminating pathogenic factors. The formula used is *Sì Jūn Zǐ Tāng* (Four Gentlemen Decoction, 四君子汤) with the addition of *shēng dì* (Radix Rehmanniae), *zǐ huā dì dīng* (Herba Violae), *zǐ cǎo* (Radix Arnebiae seu Lithospermi), and *bǎn lán gēn* (Radix Isatidis).

Arhythmia can be treated by opening yang, invigorating the blood, and draining water, as well as clearing heat, in order to remove toxin. Since retention of water, blood, phlegm, and food all affect the rhythm of the heart, herbs for invigorating the blood and draining water are used. *Dāng Guī Sháo Yào Sǎn* (Chinese Angelica and Peony Powder) is used together with *Guā Lóu Xiè Bái Bái Jiǔ Tāng* (Trichosanthes, Chinese Chive and White Wine Decoction), with *guì zhī* (Ramulus Cinnamomi), *pú gōng yīng* (Herba Taraxaci), *chuān huáng lián* (Rhizoma Coptidis from Sichuan Province of China) and *gān cǎo* (Radix Glycyrrhizae).

Joint pain can be treated by dredging the collaterals, eliminating blockage, and removing toxin. The formula used is *Shēng Mài Sǎn* (Pulse Engendering Powder) in order to nourish the heart yin. For dredging the collaterals and eliminating blockage, *Xuān Bì Tāng* (Painful Obstruction Resolving Decoction), mentioned in the *Wēn Bìng Tiáo Biàn* (Explanation of Warm Disease, 温病条辨) can be used. For removing toxin, *jīn yín huā* (Flos Lonicerae) and *dà qīng yè* (Folium Isatidis, 大青叶) can be added.

Chronic low-grade fever and aversion to cold can be treated by *Chái Hú Guì Zhī Tāng* (Bupleurum and Cinnamon Twig Decoction) for regulating nutrient qi and defensive qi. Regulating the nutrient qi and defensive qi is the key method for adjusting body temperature. *Guì zhī* (Ramulus Cinnamomi) and *gān cǎo* (Radix Glycyrrhizae) are sweet and acrid, so can transform yang; *sháo yào* (Chinese herbaceoous peony) and *gān cǎo* (Radix Glycyrrhizae) are sour and sweet, so can transform yin. *Shēng jiāng* (Ginger) strengthens yang and *dà zǎo* (Jujube) supports yin.

Chái hú (Radix Bupleuri), *rén shēn* (Radix Ginseng), *bàn xià* (Rhizoma Pinelliae) and *huáng qín* (Radix Scutellariae) can strengthen the effect of regulating nutrient qi and defensive qi.

〖 Case Study 〗

[Case 1]

Niu, 7 years old, came to the hospital in 1976 because of fever and secondary myocarditis. After leaving the hospital, she still suffered from tidal fever, palpitations, shortness of breath, and rapid, thin and weak pulse. The treatment method was to nourish yin, clear heat, remove toxin, and open yang.

[Formula]

Chinese Name	Pin Yin	Amount	Latin Name
沙参	*shā shēn*	18g	Radix Adenophorae Strictae
麦冬	*mài dōng*	12g	Radix Ophiopogonis
五味子	*wǔ wèi zǐ*	9g	Fructus Schizandrae
生地	*shēng dì*	12g	Radix Rehmanniae
蒲公英	*pú gōng yīng*	30g	Herba Taraxaci
金银花	*jīn yín huā*	15g	Flos Lonicerae
紫花地丁	*zǐ huā dì dīng*	9g	Herba Violae
栝蒌	*guā lóu*	18g	Fructus Trichosanthis
薤白	*xiè bái*	9g	Bulbus Allii Macrostami
半夏	*bàn xià*	12g	Rhizoma Pinelliae
甘草	*gān cǎo*	9g	Radix Glycyrrhizae
生石膏	*shēng shí gāo*	15g	Gypsum Fbrosum

10 doses.

[The second visit]

The fever was reduced, her pulse was relatively moderate, and she had slight edema. The formula used was *Shēng Mài Sǎn* (Pulse Engendering Powder) and *Má Xìng Shí Gān Tāng* (Ephedra, Apricot Kernel, Gypsum and Licorice Decoction, 麻杏石甘汤) combined with *bǎn lán gēn* (Radix Isatidis), *pú gōng yīng* (Herba Taraxaci), *jīn yín huā* (Flos Lonicerae) and *shēng dì* (Radix Rehmanniae) added; 10 doses.

[The third visit]

The cough stopped, but there were still palpitations, tidal fever, and rapid and weak pulse. The formula prescribed before was used, minus the *shí gāo* (Gypsum Fibrosum) and with the addition of *huáng lián* (Rhizoma Coptidis) powder 0.9g.

[The fourth visit]

The pulse was moderate and not intermittent, but there was still tidal fever. The previous formula was used with the addition of *jié gěng* (Herba Schizonepetae) 9g.

[The fifth visit]

The pulse was rapid and weak. *Yuè Bì Tāng* (Maidservant From Yue Decoction) was used with the addition of *jīn yín huā* (Flos Lonicerae), *pú gōng yīng* (Herba Taraxaci), *bǎn lán gēn* (Radix Isatidis) and *dà zǎo* (Fructus Jujubae). Five doses.

[The sixth visit]

There was slight fever, dry stool, and rapid pulse. The previous formula was used, with 1.5g of *Zǐ Xuě Dān* (Purple Snow Elixir, 紫雪丹) added (to be put into boiled water before being taken).

[The seventh visit]

The fever was gone, rapid and weak pulse, and pale tongue. *Shēng*

Mài Sǎn (Pulse Engendering Powder) was used together with *Dāng Guī Bǔ Xuè Tāng* (Chinese Angelica blood Supplementing Decoction), with the addition of herbs for clearing heat and removing toxin. *Wǔ wèi zǐ* (Fructus Schizandrae) 9g; *mài dōng* (Radix Ophiopogonis) 15g; *shā shēn* (Radix Adenophorae Strictae) 18g; *shēng dì* (Radix Rehmanniae) 12g; *zhì gān cǎo* (Radix Glycyrrhizae Preparata) 9g; *dāng guī* (Radix Angelicae Sinensis) 6g; *huáng qí* (Radix Astragali) 9g; *jīn yín huā* (Flos Lonicerae) 15g; *pú gōng yīng* (Herba Taraxaci) 18g; *zǐ huā dì dīng* (Herba Violae) 9g; *shí chāng pú* (Rhizoma Acori Tatarinowii, 石菖蒲) 6g; Five doses.

After half a year of treatment, the patient was cured.

[Case 2]

Jiang, female, 15 years old. In October 1975 she was hospitalized because of myocarditis due to Wind-Damp disease. She was discharged from the hospital five weeks later. After that she suffered from low fever, palpitations, shortness of breath, fatigue, thin and rapid pulse. The treatment focused on tonifying the heart, nourishing yin, clearing heat, and removing toxin:

Chinese Name	Pin Yin	Amount	Latin Name
生地	*shēng dì*	9g	Radix Rehmanniae
麦冬	*mài dōng*	18g	Radix Ophiopogonis
沙参	*shā shēn*	30g	Radix Adenophorae Strictae
甘草	*gān cǎo*	9g	Radix Glycyrrhizae
茯苓	*fú líng*	12g	Poria
杏仁	*xìng rén*	9g	Semen Armeniacae Amarum
蒲公英	*pú gōng yīng*	30g	Herba Taraxaci
金银花	*jīn yín huā*	9g	Flos Lonicerae
紫花地丁	*zǐ huā dì dīng*	12g	Herba Violae
远志	*yuǎn zhì*	9g	Radix Polygalae
酸枣仁	*suān zǎo rén*	9g	Semen Jujubae

After taking 30 doses of the formula, over 3 months, the patient was cured.

[Case 3]

Cao, female, 37 years old. After catching cold, she began to suffer from chest oppression with slight pain and a heart rate of 110 beats per minute. In February 1975, she came to the hospital. Her pulse then was deep, slow, and weak, with one skip every three pulses. The formula used first was *Guì Zhī Jiā Sháo Yào Tāng* (Cinnamon Twig Decoction Plus Peony, 桂枝加芍药汤) combined with *Dāng Guī Sháo Yào Sǎn* (Chinese Angelica and Peony Powder) and *pú gōng yīng* (Herba Taraxaci, 蒲公英), in order to open yang, invigorate the blood, drain water, regulate nutrient qi and defensive qi, clear heat and remove toxins:

Chinese Name	Pin Yin	Amount	Latin Name
茯苓	*fú líng*	12g	Poria
白术	*bái zhú*	9g	Rhizoma Atractylodis Macrocephalae
泽泻	*zé xiè*	18g	Rhizoma Alismatis
当归	*dāng guī*	9g	Radix Angelicae Sinensis
白芍	*bái sháo*	15g	Radix Paeoniae Alba
川芎	*chuān xiōng*	9g	Rhizoma Chuanxiong
蒲公英	*pú gōng yīng*	30g	Herba Taraxaci
甘草	*gān cǎo*	9g	Radix Glycyrrhizae
桂枝	*guì zhī*	9g	Ramulus Cinnamomi
生姜	*shēng jiāng*	9g	Rhizoma Zingiberis Recens
大枣	*dà zǎo*	7 pieces	Fructus Jujubae

Ten doses.

[The second visit]

March 17. After taking the medicine, all the symptoms were slightly improved. The previous formula was used, with the deletion of *guì zhī*

(Ramulus Cinnamomi), *shēng jiāng* (Rhizoma Zingiberis Recens), and *dà zǎo* (Fructus Jujubae). At the same time, *Guā Lóu Xiè Bái Bái Jiǔ Tāng* (Trichosanthes, Chinese Chive and White Wine Decoction) was also used, with the addition of *dǎng shēn* (Radix Codonopsis) 30g. After taking ten doses, the patient's condition was significantly improved. After taking ten more doses of the two formulas, the patient was cured.

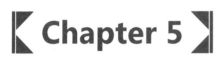

Chapter 5

Brief Comments on Slow Pulse

Slow pulse means a pulse that beats three times within one respiration. This indicates an insufficiency of yang qi and a problem of cold. According to the *Shāng Hán Lùn* (On Cold Damage) , a slow pulse may indicate jaundice, or a *Sì Nì Tāng* (Frigid Extremities Decoction) pattern, or a *Guì Zhī Tāng* (Cinnamon Twig Decoction) pattern, or a *Dà Chéng Qì Tāng* (Major Purgative Decoction, 大承气汤) pattern. This idea has been over-looked by many doctors who have studied the *Shāng Hán Lùn*. The *Líng Shū* (Spiritual Pivot) says that "*salty taste enters the blood and excessive salty food causes thirst. When entering the stomach, the effect of salty taste moves upwards into the middle jiao, flows into the channels and enters the blood and qi. When entering into the blood, the salty taste causes blood stagnation. When the blood is stagnant, the fluid in the stomach will flow into the vessels. This is why it causes thirst.*" In the *Shāng Hán Lùn*, the patterns to be treated by *Dà Chéng Qì Tāng* (Major Purgative Decoction), *Xiǎo Chéng Qì Tāng* (Minor Purgative Decoction, 小承气汤), and *Má Zǐ Rén Wán* (Cannabis Fruit Pill, 麻子仁丸) are all due to consumption of the body fluid by heat. If the consumption is severe, the vessels will be seriously affected. The pattern treated by *Xiǎo Chéng Qì Tāng* (Minor Purgative Decoction) has not transformed into dryness yet, so the consumption of fluid is not severe; that is why the pulse is slippery. In the pattern treated by *Dà Chéng Qì Tāng* (Major Purgative Decoction), dry feces have already formed, so the fluid is consumed. That is why the pulse is slow. In the pattern treated by *Má Zǐ Rén Wán* (Cannabis Fruit Pill), both the stomach fluids and the spleen fluids are damaged, so the pulse is not only slow, but also choppy. In all three patterns, there is constipation, but the pulse is different. Therefore, the treatment methods used are different. It is important to preserve body fluid in treating *yangming* diseases.

There is another kind of slow pulse that is not caused by cold, orphlegm, abdominal masses, or a *yangming* pattern. The clinical manifestations are chest oppression, shortness of breath, palpitations, and a slow pulse. Although the manifestations are related to the heart, the cause of the disease is in fact in the kidney. The pulse originates from the kidney and is related to the stomach, heart, lung, and liver. In the pattern of palpitations treated by *Zhì Gān Cǎo Tāng* (Honey-Fried Licorice Decoction), the pulse is knotted and intermittent; in the pattern of fainting and diarrheatreated by *Sì Nì Tāng* (Frigid Extremities Decoction), the pulse is fine and thin. In the pattern of shortness of breath and palpitations treated by *Shēng Mài Sǎn* (Pulse Engendering Powderr), the pulse is rapid and weak. Therefore, for this pattern, *Jīn Guì Shèn Qì Wán* (Golden Coffer Kidney Qi Pill, 金匮肾气丸), *Zhì Gān Cǎo Tāng* (Honey-Fried Licorice Decoction), *Shēng Mài Sǎn* (Pulse Engendering Powder), *Èr Xiān Tāng* (Two Immortals Decoction, 二仙汤), and *Bǎo Yuán Tāng* (Original Qi Preserving Decoction, 保元汤) are often used with modifications. The kidney stores the essence of the five *zang* organs and six *fu* organs. When the kidney-qi is insufficient, it cannot provide essence for the heart. That is why the pulse is slow and there appears chest oppression, palpitations, and shortness of breath.

〖 Chapter 6 〗

Treatment of Congestive Heart Failure with *Zhēn Wǔ Tāng* (True Warrior Decoction) Combined with the Three Methods Used to Treat Edema

Congestive heart failure is a symptom in various heart diseases. I often treat it with *Zhēn Wǔ Tāng* (True Warrior Decoction) combined with the three methods used to treat edema.

The heart stores the spirit and houses the vessels. The blood flows along certain definite directions, so reverse flow will cause disease. When heart yang is vigorous, the blood in the heart will be sufficient. If the blood flows abnormally, blood stagnation will be caused, leading to swelling, distension, and ascites. The *Jīn Guì Yào Lüè* (Essential Prescriptions of the Golden Coffer) says that edema caused by a blood disorder is called blood-Separation, while a blood disorder caused by edema is called Water-Separation, indicating the close relationship between edema and blood disorders. In the *Huáng Dì Nèi Jīng* (Yellow Emperor's Inner Canon), the saying of *"removing stagnation"* means dredging the vessels, the saying of *"opening the sweat pores"* means promoting the flow of lung qi, the saying of *"empting the urinary bladder"* means draining urine. When these three methods are used, edema should be eliminated, but why does it relapse again? This is because such a treatment only focuses on the secondary aspects of the disease. In order to deal with such a disease, the treatment should concentrate on strengthening the heart, warming the kidney, and draining water.

In the clinic, heart failure patients usually have deficiency of both the heart and the kidney, and can be treated by *Zhēn Wǔ Tāng* (True Warrior Decoction) in order to strengthen the heart yang, eliminate obstruction, and drain water. Pulmonary blood stasis, hepatomegaly, and edema in heart failure suggest a decline of heart yang, stagnation of lung qi, blood stasis, and failure of water to transform qi. To deal with such problems, *Zhēn Wǔ Tāng* (True Warrior Decoction) should be used together with the three methods to treat edema.

〖 Case Study 〗

〖 Case 1 〗

Heart disease with hypertension and heart failure. Pattern differentiation: Decline of heart yang, reverse flow of water due to yang deficiency attacking the heart and lung, and stagnation of lung qi. *Zhēn Wǔ Tāng* (True Warrior Decoction) was used as the main formula, and at the same time, the therapeutic method for opening sweat pores was also used. Digitalis was not used.

〖 Case 2 〗

Chronic cor pulmonale and heart failure. Pattern differentiation: yang deficiency in the heart and kidney, and stagnation of lung qi. *Zhēn Wǔ Tāng* (True Warrior Decoction) was used together with *Yuè Bì Tāng* (Maidservant From Yue Decoction). Digitalis was not used.

Comments

The method of empting the urinary bladder was used to promote the flow of water in order to eliminate edema. If there are symptoms of heart failure, ascites, and severe difficulty in urination, *Wǔ Líng Sǎn* (Five Substances Powder with Poria, 五苓散) can be used with the addition of *chē qián zǐ* (Semen Plantaginis) (wrapped up before being decocted) 15g; *chén xiāng* (Lignum Aquilariae Resinatum) 9g, and *ròu guì* (Cotex Cinnamomi) 9g (added at the end). This is actually modified *Xiāo Shuǐ Shèng Yù Tāng* (Reduce Water to Sagely Cure Decoction), which is composed of *Guì Zhī Tāng* (Cinnamon Twig Decoction), with the subtraction of *sháo yào* (Chinese herbaceoous peony) and the addition of *Má Huáng Fù Zǐ Xì Xīn Tāng* (Ephedra, Aconite and Asarum Decoction, 麻黄附子细辛汤) with the addition of *zhī mǔ* (Rhizoma Anemarrhenae) and *fáng jǐ* (Radix Stephaniae Tetrandrae).

[Case 3]

Chronic cor pulmonale and heart failure. Pattern differentiation: yang deficiency in the heart and kidney, and stagnation of phlegm and dampness. The treatment focused on warming yang and draining water. The formula used was *Xiāo Shuǐ Shèng Yù Tāng* (Reduce Water to Sagely Cure Decoction). Digitalis was not used. Within thirteen days, the heart failure was under control.

Comments

The method for removing stagnation mentioned in the *Huáng Dì Nèi Jīng* (Yellow Emperor's Inner Canon) is for eliminating abdominal masses, dredging the collaterals, and activating the blood to resolve stasis.

Cyanosis, hepatomegaly, and increased venous pressure in heart failure all indicate blood stasis. That is why heart failure and blood stasis are often followed by edema. The ideas of blood-Separation and Water-Separation mentioned in the *Jīn Guì Yào Lüè* (Essential Prescriptions of the Golden Coffer) suggest two conditions. One is deficiency of both blood and qi. The other is stagnation of turbid substance, with symptoms such as chest oppression, panting, cough, and enlargement of the liver and spleen in congestive heart failure. To deal with such problems, *Zhēn Wǔ Tāng* (True Warrior Decoction) should be used together with the method for removing stagnation, such as *Táo Hóng Sì Wù Tāng* (Peach Kernel and Carthamus Four Substances Decoction, 桃红四物汤), with the deletion of *shēng dì* (Radix Rehmanniae) and the addition of *ǒu jié* (Nodus Nelumbinis) and *sū mù* (Lignum Sappan).

[Case 4]

Song, female, 38 years old, suffered from mitral stenosis and congestive heart failure due to rheumatic heart disease. *Zhēn Wǔ Tāng* (True Warrior Decoction) was used together with the method for removing stagnation. After treatment, urination increased. When this treatment was stopped, the condition of the patient became worsened and urine was markedly reduced. The previous method was used again, and the condition of the patient was controlled.

Comments

I treated another patient with heart disease due to syphilis and congestive heart failure. After hospitalization, his heart failure was controlled, but it recurred after catching cold. The manifestations then were unbearable pain in the liver region, cough, palpitations, and continuous sweating. The method for removing stagnation was used together with *Yù Píng Fēng Sǎn* (Jade Wind-Barrier Powder, 玉屏风散). After one month of treatment, all the symptoms were improved.

According to the *Jīn Guì Yào Lüè* (Essential Prescriptions of the Golden Coffer), water, qi, and blood are closely related to each other. So a blood disorder can be treated from the water aspect and vice versa. Qi can be transformed by warming; blood can be activated by warming, and water and be moved by warming. That was why herbs like *ròu guì* (Cotex Cinnamomi) and *chén xiāng* (Lignum Aquilariae Resinatum) were added to the main formula. If it is complicated by yin deficiency in the heart and lung, it may cause shortness of breath, cough, spontaneous sweating, decline of heart-blood, vexation, and palpitations, which can be treated with the addition of *Shēng Mài Sǎn* (Pulse Engendering Powder).

[Case 5]

Xie, male, 45 years old, suffered from heart disease with heart failure. The clinical manifestations were cough, panting, palpitations, and inability to sit straight or lie down. *Zhēn Wǔ Tāng* (True Warrior Decoction) combined with *Shēng Mài Sǎn* (Pulse Engendering Powder) was used.

Comments

Heart failure is often marked by arrhythmia. To deal with this, we usually use *Zhì Gān Cǎo Tāng* (Honey-Fried Licorice Decoction), *Guì Zhī Gān Cǎo Lóng Gǔ Mǔ Lì Tāng* (Cinnamon Twig, Licorice, Os Draconis and Ostrea Decoction, 桂枝甘草龙骨牡蛎汤), and *Fú Líng Gān Cǎo Tāng* (Poria and Licorice Decoction, 茯苓甘草汤). To treat yin deficiency, *Zhì Gān Cǎo Tāng* (Honey-Fried Licorice Decoction) can be used together with *Shēng Mài Sǎn* (Pulse Engendering Powder). To treat yang deficiency, *Zhēn Wǔ Tāng* (True Warrior Decoction) can be used with heavy dosage. To cope with agitation and palpitations due to water harassing the heart, *Guì Zhī Lóng Gǔ Mǔ Lì Tāng* (Cinnamon Twig, Os Draconis and Ostrea Decoction, 桂枝龙骨牡蛎汤) can be used. In treating heart failure, the formulas mentioned above also can be used to deal with arrhythmia.

(All 5 cases below were treated only with Chinese Herbs)

[Case 6]

Dong, female, 56 years old, married, peasant in Beijing, suffered from cough for three months with shortness of breath and palpitations. On December 28, 1963 she was hospitalized.The patient suffered from cough and panting for over 20 years, but these symptoms could be alleviated spontaneously and the patient could work normally. She went to the hospital several times, but this did not help. In the most recent 5-6 years, she coughed frequently, and when it was severe, she was completely bed-ridden. Three days before hospitalization, her condition worsened. The manifestations were cough, dyspnea, vomiting of frothy white sputum, inability to lie down, severe cough at night, reduced appetite, upper abdominal distension and fullness, thirst, and no desire to drink water. History: enlarged mass in the neck for 30 years.

[Physical examination]

Flushed complexion, cyanosis, body temperature 36℃, blood pressure 180/120 mmHg, distention of the jugular veins, enlargement of the thyroid gland, dry sound in the lungs, apex beat in the fifth and sixth costal regions, heart rate 180 times per minute, mild blowing, systolic murmur, second sound of aortic area, softness of abdomen, ascites, and edema in the lower limbs.

[Pattern differentiation]

The manifestations were cough, dyspnea, vomiting of frothy white sputum, inability to lie down, severe cough at night, reduced appetite, upper abdominal distension and fullness, thirst and no desire to drink water. Pulse: thin, rapid, and weak. Tongue: thin and white tongue coating, pale body. The kidney is the root of qi and the location of the Life-Gate (Ming Men). If kidney yang is deficient, water cannot be controlled and flows adversely upwards to prevent lung qi from descending. Cough, panting, palpitations, inability to lie down, scanty urine, and edema of the limbs all indicate decline of heart yang. Therefore, the treatment should focus on warming yang, promoting the flow of water, nourishing the heart and diffusing the lung, and strengthening yang to eliminate stagnation. The formulas used were *Zhēn Wǔ Tāng* (True Warrior Decoction), *Shēng Mài Sǎn* (Pulse Engendering Powder), and *Yuè Bì Tāng* (Maidservant From Yue Decoction) with modification.

[Process of treatment]

1. Since there were symptoms of phlegm and dampness stagnation,

failure of lung qi to disperse, and weakness of heart yang, *Zhēn Wǔ Tāng* (True Warrior Decoction), *Yuè Bì Tāng* (Maidservant From Yue Decoction), and *Shēng Mài Sǎn* (Pulse Engendering Powder) were used with modification.

[Formula]

Chinese Name	Pin Yin	Amount	Latin Name
黑附片	*hēi fù piàn*	9g	Radix Aconiti lateralis Preparata
杭芍药	*háng sháo yào*	12g	Radix Paeoniae Alba
生姜	*shēng jiāng*	9g	Rhizoma Zingiberis Recens
大枣	*dà zǎo*	6 pieces	Fructus Jujubae
党参	*dǎng shēn*	18g	Radix Codonopsis
麦冬	*mài dōng*	12g	Radix Ophiopogonis
五味子	*wǔ wèi zǐ*	6g	Fructus Schizandrae
鲜白茅根	*xiān bái máo gēn*	60g	Fresh Rhizoma Imperatae
生石膏	*shēng shí gāo*	15g	Gypsum Fbrosum
麻黄	*má huáng*	4.5g	Herba Ephedrae
甘草	*gān cǎo*	9g	Radix Glycyrrhizae
云苓	*yún líng*	15g	Poria from Yunnan Province of China
白术	*bái zhú*	9g	Rhizoma Atractylodis Macrocephalae

In addition to taking the medicines prescribed, the patient was also provided with oxygen. After taking two doses of the formula, the symptoms of panting, cough, and shortness of breath were alleviated, sleep at night was improved, and paroxysmal dyspnea at night was reduced. But the chest fullness and distress remained unchanged, and the blood pressure was 170/120mmHg. Herbs for activating the blood, regulating qi, and calming the Spirit were added to the previous formula, such as *sū mù* (Lignum Sappan) 12g; *zhǐ qiào* (Fructus Aurantii) 6g; *lóng gǔ* (Os Draconis), and *mǔ lì* (Concha Ostreae) 15g each.

2. Nineteen days after being hospitalized, the panting stopped, the patient could perform normal activities, and the heart rate was reduced to 90 beats per minute. The remaining symptoms were stomach

distension, headache, and epigastric focal distension. The blood pressure was 180/130mmHg. Then herbs for promoting yang, removing blockage, eliminating dampness and resolving phlegm were used.

[Formula]

Chinese Name	Pin Yin	Amount	Latin Name
全栝蒌	quán guā lóu	30g	Fructus Trichosanthis
薤白	xiè bái	12g	Bulbus Allii Macrostami
半夏	bàn xià	12g	Rhizoma Pinelliae
云苓	yún líng	12g	Poria from Yunnan Province of China
陈皮	chén pí	9g	Pericarpium Citri Reticulatae
枳实	zhǐ shí	6g	Fructus Aurantii Immaturus
竹茹	zhú rú	12g	Caulis Bambusae in Taeniam
丹参	dān shēn	12g	Radix Salviae Miltiorrhizae
杜仲	dù zhòng	12g	Cortex Eucommiae
桑寄生	sāng jì shēng	30g	Herba Taxilli
牛膝	niú xī	12g	Radix Achyranthis Bidentatae

3. After taking two doses of the previous formula, the patient caught a cold and began to have a headache, stiff neck, and hypochondriac fullness. Then herbs for harmonizing and releasing were used:

Chinese Name	Pin Yin	Amount	Latin Name
桑寄生	sāng jì shēng	30g	Herba Taxilli
钩藤	gōu téng	12g	Ramulus Uncariae Cumuncis
白薇	bái wēi	12g	Radix et Rhizoma Cynanchi Atrati
菊花	jú huā	12g	Flos Chrysanthemi
柴胡	chái hú	12g	Radix Bupleuri
葛根	gé gēn	18g	Radix Puerariae
半夏	bàn xià	9g	Rhizoma Pinelliae
枳壳	zhǐ qiào	6g	Fructus Aurantii
杭芍药	háng sháo yào	9g	Radix Paeoniae Alba
甘草	gān cǎo	6g	Radix Glycyrrhizae

4. After taking two more doses of the previous formula, the superficial pattern was relieved and there were no palpitations, shortness of breath, nor epigastric focal distention. The patient could leave bed, do some activities, and desired to have food. X-ray showed that the heart shadow was reduced, stagnation of blood in the lungs was alleviated and pleural effusion disappeared.

[Case 7]

Deng, female, 48 years old, married, housewife from Hebei Province, was hospitalized on June 15, 1963.

The patient suffered from edema for half a year. In the previous week her condition worsened. In January 1961 she caught a cold and began to suffer from cough, shortness of breath, and lower limbs edema. After treatment, her problem was improved but she often had palpitations, which became severe two months ago, accompanied by shortness of breath, lower limb edema, epigastric focal distention, cough, vomiting of white sputum, and scanty urine.

[Physical examination]

Sits up straight for breathing, facial edema, mild cyanosis of the lips, distention of the jugular veins, enlargement of the left side of the heart, the heart rate of 100 beats per minute and blowing systolic murmur; sonorous echo in percussing the chest, thin and wet sound in the lungs; slight bulge of the abdomen and shifting dullness.

[Diagnosis]

Chronic bronchitis, obstructive emphysema, chronic cor pulmonale, heart failure.

[Pattern differentiation]

Yang deficiency in the heart and kidney, stagnation of phlegm and dampness, and blockage of lung qi. *Zhēn Wǔ Tāng* (True Warrior Decoction) should be used together with the method for opening sweat pores and warming yang, releasing lung qi, expelling phlegm, and draining dampness.

[Formula]

Chinese Name	Pin Yin	Amount	Latin Name
附子	*fù zǐ*	6g	Radix Aconiti Lateralis Preparata
杭芍药	*háng sháo yào*	9g	Radix Paeoniae Alba
白术	*bái zhú*	9g	Rhizoma Atractylodis Macrocephalae
云苓	*yún líng*	12g	Poria from Yunnan Province of China
甘草	*gān cǎo*	9g	Radix Glycyrrhizae
麻黄	*má huáng*	3g	Herba Ephedrae
生石膏	*shēng shí gāo*	12g	Gypsum Fbrosum
生姜	*shēng jiāng*	9g	Rhizoma Zingiberis Recens
杏仁	*xìng rén*	9g	Semen Armeniacae Amarum
白茅根	*bái máo gēn*	30g	Rhizoma Imperatae
车前子	*chē qián zǐ*	15g	Semen Plantaginis (wrapped up before being decocted)
大枣	*dà zǎo*	5 pieces	Fructus Jujubae

After taking three doses of the formula, the amount of urine was increased, 1500-1900ml a day, and lower limb edema was significantly improved. After taking the fifth dose, the cough was improved and only the calves were slightly swollen. Then herbs for soothing the chest and regulating qi were added, such as *hòu pò* (Cortex Magnoliae Officinalis) 6g and *chén pí* (Pericarpium Citri Reticulatae) 6g. After taking the sixth dose, the edema disappeared, the heart rate was slowed, and a wet noise could be heard from the lungs. The remaining symptoms were chest oppression, cough, and shortness of breath. The previous formula was used with the deletion of *bái máo gēn* (Rhizoma Imperatae), *hòu pò* (Cortex Magnoliae Officinalis), and *chē qián zǐ* (Semen Plantaginis). *Sū zǐ* (Fructus Perillae)

9g, was addeds, for stopping cough and descending qi. After taking five more doses, the cough stopped and the remaining symptoms were slight panting and mild epigastric focal distention. Then *Hòu Pò Má Huáng Tāng* (Officinal Magnolia Bark and Ephedra Decoction) was used for reducing heat, expelling phlegm, and stopping cough. One week after taking the medicines prescribed, all the symptoms were eliminated.

[Case 8]

Zhang, male, 54 years old, worker in Hebei Province, married.

The patient suffered from cough and dyspnea for 5 years. In the most recent two weeks, his problems worsened. The patient was hospitalized in November 1961 because of cough and dyspnea. The diagnosis then was cor pulmonale heart failure. After taking both Chinese and Western medicine, the heart failure was controlled. This time his cough and dyspnea worsened because of a cold, with the symptoms of excessive sticky sputum, edema of the limbs, scanty urine, epigastric focal distention, and abdominal distension.

[Physical examination]

Morbid complexion, inability to lie down, cyanotic lips, wet noise in the lungs, heart rate of 100 beats per minute, slight enlargement of the left side of the heart, bulge of the abdomen, shifting dullness, lower limb edema, wiry, slippery and rapid pulse, white and greasy tongue coating.

[Diagnosis]

Chronic bronchitis, obstructive emphysema, chronic cor pulmonale, heart failure.

[Treatment]

According to Chinese medicine pattern differentiation, this pattern was due to yang deficiency in the heart and kidney, with stagnation of phlegm and dampness. The treatment should focus on warming yang, draining water, and resolving dampness. The formula used was *Xiāo Shuǐ Shèng Yù Tāng* (Reduce Water to Sagely Cure Decoction).

[Formula]

Chinese Name	Pin Yin	Amount	Latin Name
桂枝	*guì zhī*	9g	Ramulus Cinnamomi
甘草	*gān cǎo*	9g	Radix Glycyrrhizae
麻黄	*má huáng*	4.5g	Herba Ephedrae
黑附片	*hēi fù piàn*	9g	Radix Aconiti lateralis Preparata
知母	*zhī mǔ*	9g	Rhizoma Anemarrhenae
防己	*fáng jǐ*	12g	Radix Stephaniae Tetrandrae
生姜	*shēng jiāng*	9g	Rhizoma Zingiberis Recens
杏仁	*xìng rén*	9g	Semen Armeniacae Amarum
大枣	*dà zǎo*	6 pieces	Fructus Jujubae

After taking the medicines prescribed, urination was increased to 1500-3300ml a day, the edema disappeared, and the cough, dyspnea, and vomiting were improved. On the thirteenth day, his edema was remarkably reduced, the ascites disappeared, and only the calves were slightly swollen. His body weight was reduced from 71 kilograms to 59 kilograms. Then herbs for invigorating qi, nourishing the heart, clearing the lungs, and transforming phlegm were used.

[Formula]

Chinese Name	Pin Yin	Amount	Latin Name
党参	*dǎng shēn*	15g	Radix Codonopsis
麦冬	*mài dōng*	12g	Radix Ophiopogonis
五味子	*wǔ wèi zǐ*	6g	Fructus Schizandrae
杏仁	*xìng rén*	9g	Semen Armeniacae Amarum
甘草	*gān cǎo*	9g	Radix Glycyrrhizae

Chinese Name	Pin Yin	Amount	Latin Name
生石膏	*shēng shí gāo*	9g	Gypsum Fbrosum
麻黄	*má huáng*	15g	Herba Ephedrae
小麦	*xiǎo mài*	30g	Fructus Tritici
远志	*yuǎn zhì*	6g	Radix Polygalae
茯苓	*fú líng*	12g	Poria

After taking three doses, the cough and dyspnea were improved, but the quantity of urine was obviously reduced and the edema became serious. Then *Xiāo Shuǐ Shèng Yù Tāng* (Reduce Water to Sagely Cure Decoction) was used with the addition of *fú líng* (Poria) 30g and *chē qián zǐ* (Semen Plantaginis) (wrapped up before being decocted) 30g. With this treatment, his urine increased, the edema disappeared, cough and dyspnea were alleviated, and appetite and spirit were improved.

[Case 9]

Wang, male, 45 years old, married, from Liaoning Province.

For four years, since 1959, he suffered from palpitations and shortness of breath. In the last half year, his symptoms had worsened. In December 1963, he was hospitalized. In 1959, he caught a cold and began to suffer from fever, rapid breathing, and inability to go up stairs. He was then treated in the hospital and diagnosed as syphilitic heart disease. After treatment, his condition improved and was able to work after leaving the hospital. In July of 1960, he suddenly had severe palpitations, shortness of breath, and edema of the lower limbs. He was hospitalized again and diagnosed as having heart failure. After treatment with digitalis and Chinese medicine, his symptoms improved. After that, his heart failure returned twice and was controlled by digitalis. In the last half a year, his symptoms had worsened, accompanied by palpitations, shortness of breath, inability to lie down, paroxymal dyspnea at night, lack of appetite, and sloppy stool 3-4 times a day. Before being hospitalized, the patient used digitalis.

[Physical examination]

Body temperature was 36℃, pulse rate was 80 beats per minute, respiration was 20 times per minute, blood pressure was 150/80 mmHg, slight malnutrition, lusterless complexion, generalized sweating, rapid breathing, no mucocutaneous hemorrhagic spots, slight edema of the eyelids, distention of the jugular veins, obvious pulsation of the carotid arteries, wet noise in the bottom left of the lung, obvious apex beat.

[Process of treatment]

Chinese medicine pattern differentiation: The symptoms of palpitations, shortness of breath, inability to lie down due to panting, rapid and wiry pulse, and moist tongue without fur indicated that this disease was due to decline of yang in the heart and the kidney, with stagnation of lung qi. The treatment should focus on warming yang to grasp qi and clearing the lung to stop panting. *Zhēn Wǔ Tāng* (True Warrior Decoction) was used, together with the method for opening sweat pores.

[Formula]

Chinese Name	Pin Yin	Amount	Latin Name
附子	*fù zǐ*	9g	Radix Aconiti Lateralis Preparata
杭芍药	*háng sháo yào*	12g	Radix Paeoniae Alba
白术	*bái zhú*	9g	Rhizoma Atractylodis Macrocephalae
麻黄	*má huáng*	6g	Herba Ephedrae
杏仁	*xìng rén*	9g	Semen Armeniacae Amarum
麦冬	*mài dōng*	12g	Radix Ophiopogonis
五味子	*wǔ wèi zǐ*	6g	Fructus Schizandrae
党参	*dǎng shēn*	30g	Radix Codonopsis
甘草	*gān cǎo*	9g	Radix Glycyrrhizae

After taking two doses of the formula, the patient could lay in a horizontal position, the paroxysmal dyspnea at night disappeared, and the palpitations were also improved. After this, digitalis, which had been used for three months, was stopped. After hospitalization for 12 days, all of the symptoms were improved, and only chest oppression and shortness of breath were still unchanged. Such a condition was due to weakness of heart yang and obstruction of qi. So the treatment should focus on promoting yang and removing obstruction. For this reason, *Guā Lóu Xiè Bái Bàn Xià Tāng* (Trichosanthes, Chinese Chive and Pinellia Decoction) was used, with the addition of other ingredients, together with *Zhēn Wǔ Tāng* (True Warrior Decoction). After being hospitalized for 5 months, the patient caught cold and his heart failure recurred. Then *Yù Píng Fēng Sǎn* (Jade Wind-Barrier Powder) was used with herbs for invigorating qi, nourishing the heart, and removing stagnation.

[Formula]

Chinese Name	Pin Yin	Amount	Latin Name
当归	*dāng guī*	9g	Radix Angelicae Sinensis
黄芪	*huáng qí*	24g	Radix Astragali
桃仁	*táo rén*	9g	Semen Persicae
红花	*hóng huā*	9g	Flos Carthami
小茴香	*xiǎo huí xiāng*	6g	Fructus Foeniculi
官桂	*guān guì*	4.5g	Cortex Cinnamomi
白术	*bái zhú*	6g	Rhizoma Atractylodis Macrocephalae
防风	*fáng fēng*	6g	Radix Saposhnikoviae
防己	*fáng jǐ*	9g	Radix Stephaniae Tetrandrae
郁金	*yù jīn*	15g	Radix Curcumae
延胡索	*yán hú suǒ*	15g	Rhizoma Corydalis
生晒参	*shēng shài shēn*	9g	Dry Radix Ginseng (decocted first)
浮小麦	*fú xiǎo mài*	30g	Fructus Tritici Levis

After taking these ingredients for one month, all the symptoms were improved and the patient could leave the bed and take some activities. There were no obvious palpitations, shortness of breath, cough, or dyspnea.

[Case 10]

You, male, 24 years old, unmarried, accountant from Hebei Province.

The patient suffered from palpitations and shortness of breath for three years, which worsened in the most recent seven months. In April 29, 1964 he was hospitalized. Physical examination made in 1960 showed rheumatic heart disease, but at that time he did not have any uncomfortable feeling, only slight palpitations after work. Since 1961, there gradually appeared the symptoms of poor appetite, gastric and abdominal distension, palpitations after activity, obvious shortness of breath, and lower limb edema. In 1962 he went to a hospital and the diagnosis was rheumatic heart disease. After treatment, his problem still recurred.

[Past medical history]

Rheumatic arthralgia.

[Physical examination]

Cyanotic lips, yellow sclera, redness of the throat, no enlargement of the tonsils, distention of the jugular veins, obvious jugular pulsationsc, dry and wet rale in the lungs, obvious enlargement of the left and right sides of the heart, apex beat diffusion, blowing systolic murmur in the apical region, diastolic murmur, and arrhythmia.

[Diagnosis]

Rheumatic heart disease, mitral stenosis inadequacy, atrial fibrillation, cardiac cirrhosis, and heart failure.

[Process of treatment]

Chinese medicine pattern differentiation: This pattern was due to yang deficiency in the heart and the kidney. That is what caused the chest oppression, shortness of breath, and Painful Chest-Obstruction. *Zhì Gān Cǎo Tāng* (Honey-Fried Licorice Decoction), *Wǔ Líng Sǎn* (Five Substances Powder with Poria), *Zhēn Wǔ Tāng* (True Warrior Decoction), *Lián Zhū Yǐn* (Double Precious Beverage, 联珠饮), and *Xiāo Shuǐ Shèng Yù Tāng* (Reduce Water to Sagely Cure Decoction) were used first, but the condition of the patient was not improved. Since there were the symptoms of epigastric focal distention, deep-colored tongue, black complexion, knotted and intermittent pulse, and scanty stool, this disease must be caused bydecline of yang in the heart and the kidney and complicated by blood stasis. Then *Zhēn Wǔ Tāng* (True Warrior Decoction) was used together with the method for removing stagnation. The curative effect was significant.

[Formula]

Chinese Name	Pin Yin	Amount	Latin Name
附子	*fù zǐ*	9g	Radix Aconiti Lateralis Preparata
杭芍药	*háng sháo yào*	30g	Radix Paeoniae Alba
云苓	*yún líng*	18g	Poria from Yunnan Province of China
白术	*bái zhú*	15g	Rhizoma Atractylodis Macrocephalae
生姜	*shēng jiāng*	9g	Rhizoma Zingiberis Recens
肉桂	*ròu guì*	6g	Cortex Cinnamomi (added at the end)
沉香	*chén xiāng*	6g	Lignum Aquilariae Resinatum (added at the end)
当归	*dāng guī*	12g	Radix Angelicae Sinensis
红花	*hóng huā*	12g	Flos Carthami
白茅根	*bái máo gēn*	30g	Rhizoma Imperatae
藕节	*ǒu jié*	10 pieces	Nodus Nelumbinis

After taking five doses of this formula, the symptoms were improved, the quantity of urine was increased from 300-500 ml/daily to 1300-1700 ml/daily, his body weight was reduced 3 kilograms, the liver enlargement was reduced and became soft. There was only occasional tachycardia and the heart failure was improved. Later on, there was a shortage of *fù zǐ* (Radix Aconiti Lateralis Preparata) and the condition of the patient fluctuated. After being treated with the previous formula, his condition was stabilized. After being discharged from the hospital, all the symptoms disappeared and his heart failure was controlled.

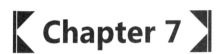

Chapter 7

Pathogenesis and Treatment of Acute and Chronic Nephritis

There are various types of nephritis. Acute nephritis may become chronic due to improper treatment. The prognosis of chronic nephritis is usually unfavourable.

How Chinese Medicine Understands Nephritis

Nephritis pertains to the concepts of "wind-water" and "edema" in Chinese medicine. According to the theory of Chinese medicine, the kidney manages storage and is closely related to the spleen and stomach. The kidney possesses both yin and yang. Kidney-Fire pertains to yang, governing the functions of reproduction and the urinary system. Kidney-Water pertains to yin, controlling the essence of the four viscera. Kidney-Fire and kidney-Water supplement and promote each other, but if kidney-Fire is excessive, kidney-Water will be damaged. Therefore, for the purpose of restoring the functions of the kidney, measures must be taken to adjust kidney-yin and kidney-yang in order to balance kidney-Water and kidney-Fire. If kidney-Fire is excessive, liver-Fire will be predominant. In this case, the liver should be purged. If kidney-yin is excessive, the spleen-yang will be deficient. In this case, the spleen should be warmed. If spleen-yang is deficienct, it will lead to an overflow of water. In this case, spleen-yang should be warmed. The spleen is the base of life after birth, and transports and transforms the essence of food and water. The spleen and kidney are intimately related, and should be closely guarded in order to sustain and support human life.

Clinically, at the early stage of nephritis, there are generally only mild symptoms of the spleen and stomach, but no obvious symptoms of yang deficiency. But if the disease is prolonged, it will lead to symptoms of spleen-yang and kidney-yang deficiency.

Clinically, there are various ideas for treating nephritis suggested by doctors in different dynasties, such as *"nourishing the kidney instead of tonifying the spleen"* and *"tonifying the spleen instead of nourishing the kidney"*. These two different ideas actually emphasize different aspects of the same problem. In the Qing Dynasty, Wang Xu-gao (王旭高) suggested that *"Weakness due to prolonged illness without abdominal mass should be treated by nourishing the kidney; if there is abdominal mass, it should be treated by tonifying the spleen"*. This understanding is obviously correct. Clinically, if symptoms of spleen and stomach yang deficiency appear, such as poor appetite, edema, sloppy stool, pale tongue, and deep, slow, or soft pulse, it should be treated by warming and tonifying the spleen yang.

The difference in treating the kidney and the spleen lies in the fact that the kidney is an organ marked by a harmonious balance between water and fire. So the herbs used to treat the kidney should not be dry, but greasy, because the kidney detests dryness and likes moistness. Meanwhile, the spleen detests dampness and likes dryness. Therefore, in the clinic, one must pay close attention to this difference and treat accordingly.

In Chinese medicine, edema is thought to be the accumulation of water. So the primary cause of edema is disease in the kidney, while its secondary cause is in the stomach. The stomach is the sea of water and grain. If the stomach is strong, it will strengthen the heart. If the heart is strengthened, it will be good for discharging urine. If urine is properly discharged, edema will be subdued.

Water is closely related to qi. So the treatment of a water problem should focus on qi. The kidney governs water and the lung is the upper source of water. So the root cause is in the kidney and the secondary cause is in the lung.

The kidney pertains to yin and the heart to yang. The kidney governs water and the heart controls the blood. Yin and yang depend on each other, while water and fire coordinate with each other. That is why herbs for activating the blood are added to the formula for promoting urination.

The symptoms of spleen and stomach weakness, severe edema, chest fullness, indigestion, sloppy stool, pale tongue, and slow pulse are caused by inactivation of spleen yang and the middle jiao being encumbered by dampness. This can be treated by warming spleen yang.

The symptoms of severe edema, normal appetite, no deficiency of the spleen and stomach yang, cold limbs, deep and slow pulse are usually caused by insufficiency of kidney yang. This should be treated by nourishing the kidney yang in order to eliminate edema.

Renal insufficiency indicates insufficiency of healthy qi (*Zhèng qì*) in the body. If healthy qi is insufficient, it will be difficult to expel pathogenic factors, and will lead to retention of waste materials in the urine. Renal insufficiency is usually marked by scanty urine or even no urine, due to insufficiency of kidney yang. To treat such a condition, drastic measures should be taken to tonify kidney yang as well as kidney yin.

The kidney is the base of life before birth while the spleen is the base of life after birth. The nutrients of food are received in the stomach, and transformed and transported by the spleen. If food does not enter the stomach, then the spleen will stop transportationation and transformation, and the kidney cannot get nourishment. Therefore, measures must be taken to protect the stomach qi during and after kidney disease.

Treatment Principles

● Eliminating pathogenic factors first in dealing with acute nephritis.

The methods for opening sweat pores and empting the urinary bladder are used to reduce edema as well as clearing heat to remove toxin. The formula to be used is *Yuè Bì Jiā Zhú Tāng* (Maidservant From Yue Decoction

Plus Atractylodes Macrocephala, 越婢加术汤) or *Má Huáng Lián Qiào Chì Xiǎo Dòu Tāng* (Herba Ephedrae, Fructus Forsythiae and Semen Phaseoli Decoction, 麻黄连翘赤小豆汤) combined with *Wǔ Líng Sǎn* (Five Substances Powder with Poria) with *bái máo gēn* (Rhizoma Imperatae) added.

The methods for clearing heat to remove toxin can be used to treat acute nephritis due to excessive heat toxin. The location of the disease is in the throat and kidney. The treatment principle is clearing heat to remove toxin. The formula to be used is *Gān Jié Tāng* (Licorice and Platycodon decoction, 甘桔汤) with the addition of *pú gōng yīng* (Herba Taraxaci), *Shān dòu gēn* (Radix Sophorae Tonkinensis, 山豆根), *niú bàng zǐ* (Fructus Arctii), *lián qiào* (Fructus Forsythiae), *xiān máo gēn* (fresh Rhizoma Imperatae) and *zhī mǔ* (Rhizoma Anemarrhenae).

Acute nephritis with anuria can be treated by *xī shuài* (Gryllus Chinensis, 蟋蟀) and *lóu gū* (Grylotalpa Africana, 蝼蛄) (3 each) (ground into powder), *chán tuì* (Periostracum Cicadae) 9g, *fú píng* (Herba Spirodelae) 9g. These ingredients are decocted, or dried and ground into a powder added to porridge with *jīng mǐ* (Oryza sativa L., 粳米), *chén pí* (Pericarpium Citri Reticulatae), *dōng guā pí* (Exocarpium Benincasae, 冬瓜皮), *xī guā pí* (Exocarpium Citrulli, 西瓜皮) and turnip.

Secondary hypertension should be treated after the heat toxin is already expelled. The herbs used are *xià kū cǎo* (Spica Prunellae, 夏枯草) 30g; *niú xī* (Radix Achyranthis Bidentatae) 18g; *cǎo jué míng* (Semen Cassiae) 30g, and *zhēn zhū mǔ* (Concha Margaritifera Usta, 珍珠母) 30g.

● Chronic nephritis should be treated by warming and nourishing the kidney Yang and tonifying the Qi and blood to restore the functions of the kidney.

Chronic nephritis may linger for years and become complicated, leading to proteinuria, low protein in the blood, swelling, ascites, pleural effusion, decline of kidney yang, scanty urine or even no urine, headache, vomiting, and uremia.

The following six methods are used with modification based on pattern differentiation:

1. Strengthening kidney yang and nourishing the kidney. For such a treatment, the dosage should be heavy. The formula used was *Shèn Qì Wán* (kidney-Qi Pill), as recorded in the *Jīn Guì Yào Lüè* (Essential Prescriptions of the Golden Coffer, 金匮要略).

[Formula]

Chinese Name	Pin Yin	Amount	Latin Name
生地	*shēng dì*	12g	Radix Rhemanniae
熟地	*shú dì*	12g	Prepared Rhizome of Rehmannia
丹皮	*dān pí*	12g	Cortex Moutan Radicis
山药	*shān yào*	18g	Rhizoma Dioscoreae
茯苓	*fú líng*	30g	Poria
泽泻	*zé xiè*	45g	Rhizoma Alismatis
山萸肉	*shān yú ròu*	12g	Fructus Corni
肉桂	*ròu guì*	9g	Cortex Cinnamomi
附子	*fù zǐ*	9g	Radix Aconiti Lateralis Preparata
菟丝子	*tù sī zǐ*	18g	Semen Cuscutae
巴戟天	*bā jǐ tiān*	15g	Radix Morindae Officinalis
淫羊藿	*yín yáng huò*	30g	Herba Epimedii
沉香	*chén xiāng*	6g	Lignum Aquilariae Resinatum (added at the end)

Chén xiāng (Lignum Aquilariae Resinatum) was added to the formula in order to guide *fù zǐ* (Radix Aconiti Lateralis Preparata) to move downwards. If there appear symptoms of reddish complexion, rapid pulse, red tongue, and yellow and scanty urine, the treatment should focus on nourishing the kidney yin. The formula used would be *Zhī Bǎi Dì Huáng Wán* (Anemarrhena, Phellodendron and Rehmannia Pill) with the addition of *bái máo gēn* (Rhizoma Imperatae), *zǐ huā dì dīng* (Herba Violae), *jīn yín huā* (Flos Lonicerae), *guī jiǎ* (Carapax et Plastrum Testudinis, 龟甲), and *ē jiāo* (Colla Corii Asini).

2. The treatment of a water problem should focus on the blood because blood stasis is the cause of edema and the result of the nephritis. The formula used is *Dāng Guī Sháo Yào Sǎn* (Chinese Angelica and Peony Powder), composed of *chuān xiōng* (Rhizoma Chuanxiong) 12g; *dāng guī* (Radix Angelicae Sinensis) 9g; *zé xiè* (Rhizoma Alismatis) 30g; *bái zhú* (Rhizoma Atractylodis Macrocephalae) 9g; *fú líng* (Poria) 15g; and *bái sháo* (Radix Paeoniae Alba) 18g; with the addition of *yì mǔ cǎo* (Herba Leonuri, 益母草) 30g; *ǒu jié* (Nodus Nelumbinis) 18g; *bái máo gēn* (Rhizoma Imperatae) 30g; and *shēng dì* (Radix Rehmanniae) 30g.

3. Prolonged illness and severe illness often damages spleen yang. Nephritis often leads to a deficiency pattern at the middle and advanced stages, characterized by pale complexion, edema of the body, weak pulse, greasy tongue coating, sloppy stool, chest distress, abdominal distension, anorexia, and aversion to cold. The treatment should first focus on warming the middle jiao. The formulas to be used are *Lǐ Zhōng Tāng* (Middle Regulating Decoction), *Xiāng Shā Liù Jūn Zǐ Tāng* (Costusroot and Amomum Six Gentlemen Decoction, 香砂六君子汤), *Píng Wèi Sǎn* (stomach Calming Powder, 平胃散), *Líng Guì Zhū Gān Tāng* (Poria, Cinnamon Twig, Atractylodes Macrocephala and Licorice Decoction), and *Chūn Zé Tāng* (Spring Pond Decoction, 春泽汤). If the disease is severe, *Fù Zǐ Lǐ Zhōng Tāng* (Middle Regulating Decoction Plus Aconite, 附子理中汤) can be used with modification. The patient should avoid eating cold or greasy food.

4. Nourishing qi and tonifying the blood: A long duration of nephritis will damage the qi and blood. The formula to be used is *Dāng Guī Bǔ Xuè Tāng* (Chinese Angelica blood Supplementing Decoction) with the addition of *lù jiǎo jiāo* (Colla Cornus Cervi), *ē jiāo* (Colla Corii Asini), or *lù róng* (Cornu Cervi Pantotrichum). The dosage of *huáng qí* (Radix Astragali) should be 60g in order to nourish qi and promote blood flow.

5. Harmonizing the liver and the stomach and descending turbid yin: during the course of nephritis, the function of the spleen and stomach

are very important. If their functions are weak, yang will not rise and yin will not descend, leading to headache, vomiting, acid regurgitation, chest fullness, no appetite and mental disorders. Non-proteinated nitrogen accumulates in the blood of some patients. To deal with such a problem, the main formula can be used together with *Wú Zhū Yú Tāng* (Evodia Decoction), with the addition of *xuán fù huā* (Flos Inulae), *dài zhě shí* (Haematitum), and *bàn xià* (Rhizoma Pinelliae). *Wú Zhū Yú Tāng* (Evodia Decoction) is composed of herbs that are warm and hot in nature, bitter and acrid in taste, and is effective for warming the liver and kidney, strengthening the source qi (Yuan qi), tranquilizing the mind, regulating the nutrient qi (*yíng qì*) and the defensive –qi (*wèi qì*).

[Formula]

Chinese Name	Pin Yin	Amount	Latin Name
吴茱萸	*wú zhū yú*	12g	Fructus Evodiae
党参	*dǎng shēn*	30g	Radix Codonopsis
生姜	*shēng jiāng*	24g	Rhizoma Zingiberis Recens
大枣	*dà zǎo*	7 pieces	Fructus Jujubae
旋覆花	*xuán fù huā*	12g	Flos Inulae
代赭石	*dài zhě shí*	18g	Haematitum
半夏	*bàn xià*	18g	Rhizoma Pinelliae

After taking the decoction, the symptoms of headache, vomiting, heartburn and acid regurgitation should disappear. The patient can then take food.

6. Treatment should focus on the primary aspect first and then on the secondary aspect.

(1) Common cold or secondary infection: such a disease often occurs and tends to recur. The formula to be used is *Yín Qiào Sǎn* (Lonicera and Forsythia Powder, 银翘散) with *chán tuì* (Periostracum Cicadae) and *fú píng* (Herba Spirodelae) added to relieve the superficial pathogenic factors. *Lú gēn* (Rhizoma Phragmitis, 芦根) and *bái máo gēn* (Rhizoma Imperatae)

are added in order to depurate the lung and cool the blood. *Pú gōng yīng* (Herba Taraxaci) and *shān dòu gēn* (Radix Sophorae Tonkinensis) are added in order to remove toxin and eliminate the focus of secondary infection. If the tonsils are red and swollen, powdered *Liù Shén Wán* (Six Spirits Pill, 六神丸) can be spread onto the tonsils.

(2) Heat production due to blood deficiency: if there are symptoms of physical weakness, night sweating, fever due to yin deficiency, and upward floating of fire, it can be treated by *Dāng Guī Liù Huáng Tāng* (Chinese Angelica Six Yellow Decoction, 当归六黄汤) with modification.

(3) Diarrhea: The treatment of diarrhea due to water-dampness attacking the lung should focus on the spleen first. The formulas to be used are *Wèi Líng Tāng* (stomach Calming Poria Decoction, 胃苓汤) and *Shēn Líng Bái Zhú Sǎn* (Ginseng, Poria and Atractylodes Macrocephala Powder, 参苓白术散) with modification. If it is caused by improper diet and infection, *Gě Gēn Huáng Qín Huáng Lián Tāng* (Pueraria, Scutellaria, and Coptis Decoction, 葛根黄芩黄连汤) can be used with modification.

● Treatment at the convalesence stage mainly focuses on supporting healthy qi and then on eliminating the remaining pathogenic factors.

Treatment at this stage still concentrates on the spleen and kidney. Once the edema and swelling have disappeared, the herbs for draining water in the formula should be reduced. If liver Fire is excessive, it should be reduced; if kidney Water is deficient, it should be nourished. With such a treatment, healthy qi will gradually be restored, and there may appear symptoms of vexation and fever. If there is no secondary infection, the fever is usually physiological, marked by vexation, fever, slight dry mouth, dry nose, low body temperature, aversion to cold and stuffy nose. The treatment at the convalescence stage should focus on nourishing the kidney yin and kidney yang. The formula to be used is *Jīn Guì Shèn*

Qì Wán (Golden Coffer Kedney Qi Pill). For nourishing the kidney-yin, *Liù Wèi Dì Huáng Wán* (Six Ingredient Rehmannia Pill) can be used. In order to strengthen the spleen, *Shēn Líng Bái Zhú Sǎn* (Ginseng, Poria and Atractylodes Macrocephala Powder) can be used. After being cured, the patient should continue to take *Shǔ Yù Wán* (Dioscorea Pill, 薯蓣丸).

● Diet:

The patient should eat vegetarian foods with a bland taste, avoiding salt. The patient should eat regularly with restricted quantity. Care should be taken to avoid overeating, overstrain, and sexual intercourse. If the complexion is improved, the edema has disappeared, and urine protein is reduced, then the patient can try to eat some salt.

Trial in taking salt: 2.5kg of salt and 2.5kg of carp are cooked together. When the water is dryed up, the carp is dryed and ground into powder for substituting salt.

● Conclusion:

1. Nephritis affects the whole body and damages the kidney, spleen, heart, and lung.

2. The treatment of nephritis at the acute stage focuses on eliminating pathogenic factors, concetrating on both the root and secondary aspects by clearing heat to remove toxin and promoting urination. If it is chronic, the treatment should focus on the root aspect for warming the kidney yang, nourishing kidney yin, strengthening the spleen, and supporting healthy qi.

3. Nephritis is complicated and tends to change. Therefore, treatment should concentrate on the main aspect and several related formulas can be used together with modification.

4. During convalescence, measures should be taken to prevent recurrence of cold attack, maintain regular diet and balance between work and rest, as well as avoid losing one's temper.

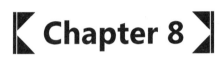

Chapter 8

Treatment of Pyelonephritis

Pyelonephritis pertains to the concept of *lín zhèng* (stranguria, 淋症) in Chinese medicine. The treatment of this disease is based on the idea of damp-heat in the bladder and deficiency of both yin and yang in the kidney.

Attack of this disease at the acute or chronic stage is often treated according to damp-heat in the lower jiao. If there are symptoms of fever, aversion to cold, painful urination, urgency in urination, slippery and rapid pulse, red tongue with a yellow and greasy tongue coating, *Bā Zhèng Sǎn* (Eight Corrections Powder, 八正散) can be used together with *Dì Fū Zǐ Tāng* (Fructus Kochiae Decoction, 地肤子汤). *Bā Zhèng Sǎn* (Eight Corrections Powder), recorded in the book entitled *Tài Píng Huì Mín Hé Jì Jú Fāng* (Imperial Grace Pharmacy Formulas, 太平惠民和剂局方), is effective for reducing heat to eliminating stranguria. *Dì Fū Zǐ Tāng* (Fructus Kochiae Decoction), recorded in the book entitled *Jì Shēng Fāng* (Life Saver Formulas, 济生方), is applicable to damp-heat in the lower jiao, with symptoms such as yellow and brown urine and unsmooth urination. *Dì fū zǐ* (Fructus Kochiae) and *shēng má* (Rhizoma Cimicifugae) are in this formula, and when combined with *Bā Zhèng Sǎn* (Eight Corrections Powder), are clinically quite significant in treating this disease. If there are excessive red blood cells in the urine, it can be treated by *Zhū Líng Tāng* (Polyporus Decoction) with the addition of *xuè yú tàn* (Crinis Carbonisatus, 血余炭), *ǒu jié* (Nodus Nelumbinis), *pú huáng* (Pollen Typhae, 蒲黄), *shēng dì* (Radix Rehmanniae), and *yì mǔ cǎo* (Herba Leonuri).

If pyelonephritis becomes chronic, it will damage yin and yang. Then the treatment should focus on clearing heat and supporting healthy qi. If there is yang deficiency, it can be treated by *Zhū Líng Tāng* (Polyporus Decoction, 猪苓汤) combined with *Guì Fù Bā Wèi Dì Huáng Wán* (Eight-Ingredient Rehmannia Pill, 桂附八味地黄丸) with the addition of *huáng qí* (Radix Astragali) and *chén xiāng* (Lignum Aquilariae Resinatum). If there is excessive fire due to yin deficiency, measures should be taken to nourishin yin and reduce fire. The formula used is *Zhī Bǎi Dì Huáng Wán* (Anemarrhena, Phellodendron and Rehmannia Pill) with the addition of herbs for removing toxin and subduing swelling. It can be treated with *Zhū Líng Tāng* (Polyporus Decoction), with the addition of *jīn yín huā* (Flos Lonicerae), *shēng dì* (Radix Rehmanniae), and *pú huáng* (Pollen Typhae); Or be treated by *Dāng Guī Sháo Yào Săn* (Chinese Angelica and Peony Powder), with the addition of *bái máo gēn* (Rhizoma Imperatae) and Che Qian Cao (Herba Plantaginis).

〖 Case Study 〗

A female patient, 30 years old, suffered from fever and lumbago, with symptoms of burning pain during urination, urgency in urination, scanty and brown urine, and rapid pulse. The tongue coating was yellow and slightly greasy, the tongue was red, and there were excessive red blood cells in her urine.

[Formula]

Chinese Name	Pin Yin	Amount	Latin Name
猪苓	zhū líng	12g	Polyporus
泽泻	zé xiè	12g	Rhizoma Alismatis
白术	bái zhú	9g	Rhizoma Atractylodis Macrocephalae
茯苓	fú líng	15g	Poria
桂枝	guì zhī	9g	Ramulus Cinnamomi
阿胶	ē jiāo	12g	Colla Corii Asini (melted into the decoction)
滑石	huá shí	12g	Talcum
甘草梢	gān cǎo shāo	6g	Tips of Radix Glycyrrhizae
生地	shēng dì	12g	Radix Rehmanniae
血余炭	xuè yú tàn	9g	Crinis Carbonisatus
地肤子	dì fū zǐ	9g	Fructus Kochiae
芍药	sháo yào	9g	Chinese herbaceoous peony

After taking five doses of this formula, all of the symptoms disappeared.

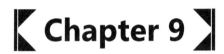

〖 Chapter 9 〗

Treatment of Diabetes Mellitus

In Chinese medicine, diabetes pertains to the "*wasting and thirsting*". This disease is mostly due to spleen and stomach yin deficiency and fire. Yang deficiency is rarely seen. Early stages of this disease are differentiated into upper, middle, and lower jiao locations, but later stages affect all three. At the early stage, treatment should focus on nourishing yin to clear heat and reduce fire. Treatment should concurrently focus on the lungs and stomach. At the middle stage, the treatment should concentrate on nourishing yin and tonifying the qi. If there are the symptoms of great hunger and thirst, be careful of excessive use of cool and cold natured herbs, since one must protect the spleen and stomach. At the advanced stage, the treatment should concentrate on the deficiency patterns involving both yin and yang.

Because a deficiency of water cannot control fire, the treatment of this disease should focus on nourishing kidney-yin. But if the deficiency of kidney-yin affects the kidney-yang, then kidney-yang also has to be taken into consideration.

The following formula is often used to deal with this disease at the middle and advanced stages:

Chinese Name	Pin Yin	Amount	Latin Name
生地	*shēng dì*	30g	unprepared Rhizome of Rehmannia
熟地	*shú dì*	30g	prepared Rhizome of Rehmannia
天冬	*tiān dōng*	12g	Radix Asparagi
麦冬	*mài dōng*	12g	Radix Ophiopogonis
党参	*dǎng shēn*	30g	Radix Codonopsis
当归	*dāng guī*	9g	Radix Angelicae Sinensis
山萸肉	*shān yú ròu*	12g	Fructus Corni
菟丝子	*tù sī zǐ*	30g	Semen Cuscutae
玄参	*xuán shēn*	12g	Radix Scrophulariae
黄芪	*huáng qí*	30g	Radix Astragali
茯苓	*fú líng*	12g	Poria
泽泻	*zé xiè*	12g	Rhizoma Alismatis

If there is excessive heat in *yangming* channel with the symptom of thirst, *Bái Hǔ Tāng* (White Tiger Decoction, 白虎汤) can be added to the main formula. *Chuān huáng lián* (Rhizoma Coptidis from Sichuan Province of China) can be used to clear heat from the stomach. Other herbs like *shí hú* (Herba Dendrobii, 石斛), *gé gēn* (Radix Puerariae), *wū méi* (Fructus Mume), and *wǔ wèi zǐ* (Fructus Schizandrae) also can be used, according to the pattern.

If there is yang deficiency at the advanced stage, *Jīn Guì Shèn Qì Wán* (Golden Coffer Kedney Qi Pill) can be used. The dosage for *guì zhī* (Ramulus Cinnamomi) and *fù zǐ* (Radix Aconiti Lateralis Preparata) is 9g. If there is abdominal distension, *hòu pò* (Cortex Magnoliae Officinalis) can be added; if there is diarrhea, the dosage of *fú líng* (Poria) and *zé xiè* (Rhizoma Alismatis) can be increased, while the dosage of *shēng dì* (Radix Rehmanniae) and *shú dì* (prepared Rhizome of Rehmannia) should be reduced. If there is hypertension, *dù zhòng* (Cortex Eucommiae) and *niú xī* (Radix Achyranthis Bidentatae) can be added. It is very important to control diet. Large dosage of *dì huáng* (Radix Rehmanniae) can reduce appetite. If there is coronary heart disease, *guā lóu* (Fructus Trichosanthis), *xiè bái* (Bulbus Allii Macrostami), and *bàn xià* (Rhizoma Pinelliae) can be added.

【 Case Study 】

Zhang, male, 49 years old, soldier.

In 1971 he was found to have diabetes mellitus. The manifestations were glucose in the urine, 232mg blood sugar, excessive eating, frequent urination, dry mouth, thirst, rapid pulse, thin and white tongue coating. Pattern differentiation was wasting and thirsting. The therapeutic methods used focused on nourishing yin, clearing heat, tonifying the qi, and promoting production of fluid.

[Formula]

Chinese Name	Pin Yin	Amount	Latin Name
生石膏	shēng shí gāo	18g	Gypsum Fbrosum
熟地	shú dì	45g	prepared Rhizome of Rehmannia
当归	dāng guī	15g	Radix Angelicae Sinensis
菟丝子	tù sī zǐ	30g	Semen Cuscutae
党参	dǎng shēn	30g	Radix Codonopsis
玄参	xuán shēn	12g	Radix Scrophulariae
枸杞子	gǒu qǐ zǐ	15g	Fructus Lycii
天冬	tiān dōng	9g	Radix Asparagi
麦冬	mài dōng	9g	Radix Ophiopogonis
川黄连	chuān huáng lián	6g	Rhizoma Coptidis from Sichuan Province of China
乌梅	wū méi	12g	Fructus Mume
泽泻	zé xiè	12g	Rhizoma Alismatis
红人参	hóng rén shēn	9g	Radix Ginseng

The patient took one dose per day. After taking 30 doses, all the symptoms disappeared. Then these ingredients were made into tablets to be taken continuously for strengthening the curative effect.

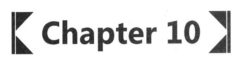

Chapter 10

Discussion on Superficial Patterns

The superficial patterns commonly encountered in clinical practice should be treated by sweating therapy. Delayed or wrong treatment will worsen the pattern.

1. Wind, cold, summer-heat, dryness, dampness, and heat are six climatic phenomena and are normally not harmful to the human body. But if human beings are not careful to avoid them under special conditions, they will become pathogenic and cause diseases. Such diseases are often characterized by aversion to cold and body pain. These diseases are exterior patterns, but are not due to exterior pathogens. Instead, they are caused by people violating the normal changes of the six climactic factors. These patterns can be cured by regulating the functions of the body and harmonizing the nutrient qi and the defensive qi. Such a treatment will induce sweating and stop fever.

2. Abnormal changes of wind, cold, summer-heat, dryness, dampness, and heat will damage all things. Under such a circumstance, people should stay at home with the doors and windows closed. Even so, diseases sometimes cannot be prevented. Once the disease has occurred, it will spread from family to family and even cause death. Such a disease is marked by manifestations of both superficial patterns and superficial pathogenic factors. Therefore, the therapeutic method used to treat it also varies. Another morbid condition is the so-called Warm Disease, which is marked by the manifestations of both superficial pattern and superficial pathogenic heat. The treatment for this should focus on clearing heat and nourishing yin because excessive heat will damage yin. If there are superificial pathogenic factors, measures should be taken to remove toxin. If heat is excessive, the blood will become turbid, therefore, yin should be nourished in order to dilute the blood. If toxin is released but not completely removed, it will damage the healthy qi. If toxin is removed but not released, then it will sink inwards. Clearing heat, nourishing yin, removing and releasing toxin will all help to cure the disease.

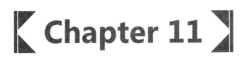

Chapter 11

Therapeutic Methods For Dealing With Fevers

Fever is a pattern, but not a disease. Fever may appear in various diseases. Therefore, the methods used to treat fever vary. Fever may be divided into two categories: endogenous and exogenous. Exogenous fever manifests in the nose while endogenous fever manifests in the mouth. The former may linger all through the course of a disease while the latter may be sometimes light and sometimes heavy. Usually, excess of yang causes fever, but deficiency of yin also can cause fever. A predominance of pathogenic factors causes an excess pattern, while an exhaustion of essence may lead to a deficiency pattern. An new disease is often excess in nature, while prolonged disease is often of a deficienct nature. Since fever may occur in various diseases, the treatment is not easy.

Human beings depend on the natural world to exist and develop. The natural world provides human beings with all the necessities, but harms the human body under special conditions. When strange substances attack the body, the body's resistance will fight against it in order to protect the body. If the body's resistance is strong enough, it will drive away the invader. If the body's resistance is not strong enough, it may fail to protect the body. The causes of diseases are various, but their effect on the nutrient qi and the defensive qi are the same.

Wind, cold, summer-heat, dryness, dampness and heat will be good to the human body when they occur at the right time in the right degree. If they occur abnormally, they can damage the body. You Zai-jing (尤在泾), a doctor in the Qing Dynasty, said: "when invisible pathogenic factors have entered the body, they will be retained in the viscera and mingle with water, blood, phlegm and food." When these invisible pathogenic factors have mingled with these turbid substances, they begin to cause abnormal changes inside the body and eventually cause diseases. When the body's resistance fights against these pathogenic factors, fever will appear. The cause of fever is never simple. So in dealing with fever, doctors have to make clear the exact cause and then concentrate the treatment on the main aspect. For example, in the pattern treated by *Xiè Xīn Tāng* (Heart Draining Decoction), epigastric focal distention is the main pattern; in the pattern treated by *Chái Hú Tāng* (Bupleurum Decoction, 柴胡汤), discomfort and fullness in the chest and hypochondria is the main pattern; In the pattern treated by *Má Huáng Tāng* (Ephedra Decoction), no sweating and aversion to cold is the main pattern; in the pattern treated by *Guì Zhī Tāng* (Cinnamon Twig Decoction), sweating and aversion to wind is the main pattern; in the pattern treated by *Gě Gēn Tāng* (Pueraria Decoction), stiffness of the back and neck is the main pattern.

In dealing with fever, care must be taken to differentiate the main pattern and the main aspect within the main pattern. For example, why is the pattern marked by diarrhea, vomiting, cold limbs, thin and indistinct pulse sometimes treated by *Sì Nì Tāng* (Frigid Extremities Decoction) and sometimes by *Wú Zhū Yú Tāng* (Evodia Decoction)? The reason for this is that in *Sì Nì Tāng* (Frigid Extremities Decoction) diarrhea is the main pattern and vomiting is the secondary pattern. In *Wú Zhū Yú Tāng* (Evodia Decoction), vomiting is the main pattern and diarrhea is the secondary pattern. The pattern treated by *Wú Zhū Yú Tāng* (Evodia Decoction) has the symptoms of fullness below the stomach, but the pattern treated by *Sì Nì Tāng* (Frigid Extremities Decoction) does not have such symptoms. In both patterns, there are the symptoms of cold limbs, thin and indistinct pulse, diarrhea, and vomiting. Fullness below the stomach only exists in the pattern treated by *Wú Zhū Yú Tāng* (Evodia Decoction). Take gastric ulcer for example: it can be treated by *Gān Cǎo Xiè Xīn Tāng* (Licorice heart Draining Decoction), *Yī Guàn Jiān* (Effective Integration Decoction), or *Xiāo Yáo Sǎn* (Free Wanderer Powder). This is because the cause of belching, acid regurgitation, borborygmus, and diarrhea lies in the stomach. That is why *Gān Cǎo Xiè Xīn Tāng* (Licorice heart Draining Decoction) is used. The cause of red tongue without coating, wiry pulse, liability to anger, and no acid regurgitation is lack of liver-yin; hence, *Yī Guàn Jiān* (Effective

Integration Decoction) is used. Excessive contemplation and working day and night will lead to liver depression. Therefore, *Xiāo Yáo Sǎn* (Free Wanderer Powder) is used. The same disease may be treated differently because of different causes. Take edema for example. If it is above the waist, the patient should be sweated; if it is below the waist, then one should disinhibit urine. That is what treating the same disease with different therapies means. In healthy people, healthy qi (*Zhèng qì*) moves regularly. If it does not move regularly, it will cause disease. The flow of healthy qi starts from *jueyin* and terminates at *taiyang*. This is regular movement. If it starts to flow from *taiyang*, it is abnormal movement. So it is very important to ensure that healthy qi moves in the right way. If it starts to flow from *jueyin*, yin and yang will be harmonized. *Chái hú* (Radix Bupleuri) is the main ingredient to guide it to flow from *jueyin*; *Guì Zhī Tāng* (Cinnamon Twig Decoction) is the formula to harmonize nutrient-qi and defensive qi. nutrient qi and defensive qi are the sources of qi and blood, while qi and blood manifest the functions of the nutrient qi and defensive qi. Both nutrient qi and defensive qi originate from the middle jiao. Hunger, overeating, and overstrain will damage the spleen and stomach, affecting the nutrient qi and defensive qi, and eventually causing fever. The formulas developed by Li Dong-yuan for supplementing the middle and tonifying qi are the main ones used to treat endogenous fever. As to the miscellaneous diseases like jaundice, malaria, sun-stroke, overstrain, and dysentery, there are special patterns and special formulas.

【 Case Study 】

In 1957, at the Beijing Children's Hospital, I treated a one year-old child who suffered from encephalitis, accompanied by high fever, unconsciousness, and convulsions. A large piece of ice was put at the side of the bed and some ice was put over the forehead of the child. Later on, wintermint was used to make the child sleep. When he woke up, convulsions attacked again and the high fever remained unchanged. I was invited for consultation. The doctors there used *Ān Gōng Niú Huáng Wán* (Peaceful Palace Bovine Bezoar Pill, 安宫牛黄丸), *Zhì Bǎo Dān* (Supreme Jewel Elixir, 至宝丹), *Zǐ Xuě Dān* (Purple Snow Elixir, 紫雪丹) and *Bái Hǔ Tāng* (White Tiger Decoction) to clear heat and remove toxin and to nourish yin in order to increase body fluids. But all these trials had failed. Examination: red tongue and restlessness. I prescribed *Huáng Qín Huáng Lián Ē Jiāo Jī Zǐ Huáng Tāng* (Radix Scutellariae, Rhizoma Coptidis, Colla Corii Asini and Vitellus Galli Decoction, 黄芩黄连阿胶鸡子黄汤). After taking this decoction, the fever disappeared and the patient was cured. A 9 year-old girl also suffered from encephalitis, with the symptoms of high fever and convulsions, but was still conscious. I used the same formula to treat her, but there was no effect. The patient had symptoms of bitter taste in the mouth, red tongue, wiry, thin, and rapid pulse. Then I used *Yī Guàn Jiān* (Effective Integration Decoction) to treat her, to good effect. Although the two cases were the same, one involved the *shaoyin*, the other involved *jueyin*. Since the location was different, the treatment also needed to be different.

Another time, a 2 year-old child suffered from fever for a long time. I was invited for consultation. The clinical manifestations were thin and weak pulse, pale complexion, pale tongue, and normal urination and defecation. This problem was caused by spleen deficiency. I used *Yín Bái Sàn* (银白散) developed by Chen Wu-ze (陈无择) and cured the patient.

A 15 year-old girl suddenly suffered from diarrhea, fever, and general weakness. Then anemia promptly occurred, with her hemoglobin dropping to 4g. Several blood transfusions did not help. After being treated in several hospitals, she returned to Beijing for treatment. The manifestations were rapid and weak pulse, poor appetite, pale complexion, mental fatigue, and weakness. I treated her with *Chái Hú Guì Zhī Tāng* (Bupleurum and Cinnamon Twig Decoction) and *Xiǎo Jiàn*

Zhōng Tāng (Minor Center Fortifying Decoction). After treatment, the fever disappeared, she could eat, and her physical condition improved. Her hemoglobin increased to 11g.

A 40 year-old man suffered from high fever (38℃) for nine years. The fever occurred once every several days and could be cured after various treatments. According to the Shang Han Lun (Treatise on Cold Diseases) theory, I used *Sì Nì Sǎn* (Frigid Extremities Powder) and *Wū Méi Wán* (Fructus Mume Pill, 乌梅丸) and cured the patient.

A 50 year-old man suffered from stomachache and diarrhea. Treatment in one hospital did not help. The manifestations were deep and weak pulse, thin and white tongue coating, epigastric focal distention, and pain. I used *Gān Cǎo Xiè Xīn Tāng* (Licorice heart Draining Decoction) to treat him. After taking three doses, the patient's body temperature was 39℃. I advised him to continue to take the formula. After the patient sweated, his fever disappeared and the stomachache stopped.

I once treated a case of pelvic inflammation with lingering high fever. After taking several doses of *Wēn Jīng Tāng* (Channel Warming Decoction, 温经汤), the fever stopped. Another woman with high fever was not cured by Western medicine. Examination revealed ulcerations on her external genitals. I diagnosed her problem as *Hú Huò* (erosion of throat, anus and genitalia) and used *Gān Cǎo Xiè Xīn Tāng* (Licorice heart Draining Decoction) to treat her. After this treatment, her fever stopped.

A 50 year-old patient suffered from lingering fever after an operation for gastric perforation. The manifestations were red tongue without coating, thirst, no sweating, no aversion to cold, constipation, and rapid and weak pulse. I used *Guī Sháo Yǐn* (Chinese Angelica and Peony Beverage, 归芍饮), adding *shēng dì* (Radix Rehmanniae) and *bái máo gēn* (Rhizoma Imperatae). After this treatment, the fever stopped.

A patient named Xiao, 9 years-old, suffered from fever, cough, headache, and sore-throat for half a month. I used acrid and cool herbs to relieve superficial pathogenic factors, but the fever was not relieved. Examination showed that his white blood cell count was 14000/mm³, his body temperature was 38℃, and the tuberculin test was negative. I was invited to treat the patient. The manifestations were white powdery tongue coating, rapid and weak pulse, and pale complexion. I prescribed three doses of *Sān Rén Tāng* (Three Kernels Decoction, 三仁汤) with modification. When the patient returned home and took the medicine at eleven o'clock, he vomited immediately. He took the medicine again in the afternoon, immediately vomited and diarrhea followed. After he took the third dose, the vomiting stopped and the fever was relieved.

〖 Chapter 12 〗

Treatment of Infantile Pneumonia Pattern

On Pneumonia Pattern

The symptoms of pneumonia, such as fever, cough, wheezing, and rhinitis can be found in many Chinese medicine classics. The manifestations of Wind-Warmth disease at the early stage are: fever, thirst, sweating, aversion to cold, and cough. If it is severe, it will transmit counter-flow into the Pericardium. As to the warm disease in winter, it is warm disease occurring in winter. Both warm disease in winter and Wind-warm diseases are newly contracted diseases due to exogenous pathogenic factors, and their patterns are similar, and both include infantile pneumonia.

On the Cause and Pathogenesis of the Disease

The cause of infantile pneumonia is exogenous. If the disease is prolonged or leads to death, it is often due to malnutrition, rickets, or congenital heart disease. This disease tends to occur in winter and spring. So the cause of the disease is either wind-cold or wind-warmth.

The cause of infantile pneumonia is largely due to stagnation of lung-qi. The *Sù Wèn* (Plain Questions) says that stagnation of qi is always related to the lung. The lung controls qi in the whole body and regulates the water passages. This is why lung-qi moves downwards. If it moves upwards, it is pathological. If it stagnates, it will cause fever, cough, dyspnea, and rhinitis. Ye Tian-shi (叶天士) said that the cause of Wind-Warmth disease was the stagnation of lung-qi that led to retention of fluid and production of phlegm. Moreover, lung disease frequently affects the heart. The heart controls the blood and the lung governs qi. If lung-qi is stagnant, the blood cannot flow smoothly, which clinically leads to pale complexion, and cyanotic lips and nails. If it is severe, it will cause heart failure. The lung opens into the nose. If lung-qi is stagnant, clear qi cannot ascend and the upper orifices will be blocked. That is what causes rhinits.

Pattern Differentiation and Diagnosis

Pneumonia is caused by invasion of pathogenic factors into the lung and reaches the blood-level. The invasion of pathogenic factors is either shallow or deep, the pathogenesis is either external transmission or internal penetration, the disease is either mild or severe, and the course is either primary or advanced. So, clinically, there are various patterns and manifestations. Generally these patterns can be divided into four types:

● Lung-heat and internal excess:

This type of pattern is caused by an invasion of warm pathogenic factors that affect the lung. The lung and the large intestine are internally and externally related to each other. If the lung shifts heat to the large intestine, then this is a *yangming* pattern, with manifestations such as stuffy, runny nose, thirst with drinking, agitation, red complexion, dry lips and nose, sweating or without sweating, cough, dyspnea, excessive sputum or yellow sticky sputum. If it is severe, there will be chest distension and fullness, mental disorder, the chest and abdomen will be very hot, constipation, scanty and brownish urine, white or yellow and dry tongue coating, deep-red tongue body, slippery and rapid pulse, or floating and rapid pulse or wiry pulse, or large and rapid pulse.

● **Excess heat injuring yin:**

This pattern is caused by pathogenic heat that obstructs the lung and consumes the body fluid, producing phlegm due to excessive heat. The phlegm will cause panting. Delayed or wrong treatment will lead to a predominance of pathogenic factors and a weakness of body resistance. The clinical manifestations are high fever, mental confusioin, ravingand unconsciousness, vexation and agitation, phlegm rales in the throat, protrusion of the chest, dyspnea, no tears and snivel, eyes staring upwards, convulsions of the limbs, neck stiffness, cold limbs, flushed or cyanotic complexion. There may be cough with excessive phlegm, fever, no sweating, severe fever in the afternoon and at night, hot soles and palms, yellow and dry or light yellow tongue coating, deep-red tongue body, thin and rapid and urgent pulse.

● **Yang deficency due to prolonged illness:**

This type is marked by weakness of the the healthy qi and lingering pathogenic factors. Pathogenic heat damages both yin and yang. If the patient has a cold consitution, the pathogenic factors tend to damage the healthy qi and consume the yang. This type of pattern is often severe. The manifestations are weak and shallow breathing, mental fatigue, cold limbs, no elevation of body temperature, thin and weak pulse and pale tongue. Sometimes heart failure also occurs.

● **Retreat of pathogenic factors and damaged healthy qi:**

This type often appears at the advanced stage when the pathogenic factors have retreated and the healthy qi has been damaged, usually characterized by weakness, low fever, light cough, lung sounds, mental fatigue, anorexia, rapid and weak pulse, palpitations after movement,/ and spontaneous sweating.

Treatment Principles for Pneumonia

Infantile pneumonia pertains to the concept of warm disease. The theory of warm disease was based on the pattern differentiation in the *Shāng Hán Lùn* (On Cold Damage). But warm disease and Cold Damage disease vary in the treatment methods. The treatment methods for Cold Damage disease are effective in inducing sweating, but ineffective in clearing heat from the nutrient (*yíng*, 营) level and removing toxin, while the methods for treating warm disease are effective for clearing heat from the nutrient level and removing toxin, but ineffective for inducing sweating. In treating warm disease, if the nutrient level is not cleared and the toxin is not removed, the fever cannot be relieved simply by sweating. If the nutrient level is cleared and the toxin is removed, but sweating is not induced, pathogenic factors cannot be eliminated and the disease will worsen.

Since pneumonia pertains to warm disease, the treatment of it should take Wei (defensive) level, qi level, Ying (Nutrient) level, and Xue (blood) level as the basis for treatment according to pattern differentiation. Ye Tian-shi suggested that is to warm disease at the defensive level, with the symptoms of fever and aversion to cold, should be treated by herbs acrid in taste and cool in nature in order to relieve pathogenic factors from the surface of the body. The dosage of the medicines should be light. Heavy dosage will guide pathogenic factors to penetrate deeper into the body. If warm disease lingers at the defensive level, it will eventually come to the qi level and cause excessive heat which can be treated by herbs acrid in taste and cold in nature to remove heat and protect body fluid. If the heat forms and congeals inside the body, herbs that are bitter, acrid and salty in taste and cold in nature should be used to open and descend qi through the stomach and intestines. If the warm disease enters the nutrient level due to failure to remove pathogenic factors at the qi level, the treatment should concentrate on clearing the nutrient level and promote qi movement. If heat is at both the qi level and the blood level, the treatment should focus on both the qi level and the nutrient level. If warm disease lingers at the blood level, it should be treated by cooling the blood and dispersing the blood. The following are the author's personal experience in treating this disease:

● The relationship between *Wei* (defensive), qi, *Ying* (Nutrient), and *Xue* (blood) levels and the treatment of pneumonia:

According to the classics, warm disease damages yin. So in treating warm diseases, acrid and cool herbs must be used together with sweet and cold herbs in order to nourish yin and cool the blood. Pneumonia pertains to warm disease and so tends to damage yin. Clinically, the duration of infantile pneumonia is often over three days. The duration of the severe cases and those that lead to death is often over five or six days. Since pneumonia involves organic pathological change of the lung, the pathogenic factors change quickly and transmit swiftly. When the disease already involves the nutrient-level and the blood-level, the treatment must focus on inducing sweating to relieve superficial pathogenic factors, clearing the nutrient-level, and removing toxin with herbs like *má huáng* (Herba Ephedrae), *xìng rén* (Semen Armeniacae Amarum), *shí gāo* (Gypsum Fibrosum), *gān cǎo* (Radix Glycyrrhizae), *lián qiào* (Fructus Forsythiae), *dān pí* (Cortex Moutan Radicis) and *shēng dì* (Radix Rehmanniae) as well as *Zhì Bǎo Dān* (Supreme Jewel Elixir) in the *Tài Píng Huì Mín Hé Jì Jú Fāng* (Imperial Grace Pharmacy Formulas, 太平惠民和剂局方).

● Treating pneumonia by taking measures before the disease has occurred:

The treatment of pneumonia based on pattern differentiation according to *Wei* (defensive-Phase), qi (defensive qi), *Ying* (nutrient-level), and *Xue* (blood level) touches on the idea that excellent doctors treat before the disease has occurred. This idea is described in the *Jīn Guì Yào Lüè* (Essential Prescriptions of the Golden Coffer), the *Nán Jīng* (Canon of Difficult Issues, 难经), and the *Líng Shū* (Spiritual Pivot). According to Chinese medicine theory and my personal clinical experience, infantile pneumonia, especially toxic pneumonia, has to be treated with preventive measures so as to prevent it from worsening. Although the clinical manifestations of pneumonia vary, the treatment principle remains the same, which is to focus on the root aspect.

If doctors can take measures to prevent the transmission of pneumonia to deeper levels, mortality will be greatly reduced. At the early stage, if *Má Xìng Shí Gān Tāng* (Ephedra, Apricot Kernel, Gypsum and Licorice Decoction) is used with the addition of acrid and cool herbs for releasing stagnated lung-qi, and other medicines like *Ān Gōng Niú Huáng* (Calculus Bovis for Calming the Uterus) or *Zhì Bǎo Dān* (Supreme Jewel Elixir) to control convulsions and unconsciousness, the disease will be controlled at the early stage and prevented from further progress.

● Joining of yin and yang and the treatment of pneumonia:

In the *Sù Wèn* (Plain Questions), the joining of yin and yang implies the fact that sweat is the yin fluid and that heat may enter the yin phase again if it cannot be relieved from the yang phase through sweating. My personal experience is that the so-called combination of yin and yang just refers to mixture between the pathogenic factors and the healthy qi.

Severe pneumonia with continuous high fever that cannot be relieved through sweating can be treated according to the idea of combination of yin and yang with the herbs acrid in taste and cool in nature for relieving heat, clearing the Nutrient-Phase, and removing toxin. Such a therapeutic method can really improve the clinic curative effect.

According to the above discussion, pneumonia pertains to warm disease due to infection of Warm toxin. Wind-Warmth disease attacks the lung first. At the early stage, warm disease damages yin. Since the location of pneumonia is in the lung and the pathogenic factors sink into the blood level, it should be treated by acrid and cool herbs in order to clear heat and remove toxin.

〖 Case Study 〗

[Case 1]

Li, one and a half years old.

The patient suffered from cough, excessive phlegm and fever for one week. The manifestations were rhinitis, panting, 39℃ body temperature, breathing 60 times per minute, listless, no sweating, thin and white tongue coating, floating and rapid pulse.

[Diagnosis]

pneumonia.

[Pattern differentiation]

Wind-Warmth attacking the lung.

[Treatment principle]

clear heat to remove toxin, release superificial pathogenic factors with acrid and cool herbs.

[Formula]

Má Xìng Shí Gān Tāng (Ephedra, Apricot Kernel, Gypsum and Licorice Decoction) with additions.

[Ingredients]

Chinese Name	Pin Yin	Amount	Latin Name
麻黄	*má huáng*	3g	Herba Ephedrae
杏仁	*xìng rén*	9g	Semen Armeniacae Amarum
甘草	*gān cǎo*	6g	Radix Glycyrrhizae
生石膏	*shēng shí gāo*	12g	Gypsum Fbrosum
金银花	*jīn yín huā*	6g	Flos Lonicerae Japonicae
连翘	*lián qiào*	9g	Fructus Forsythiae
桔梗	*jié gěng*	6g	Radix Platycodi
荆芥穗	*jīng jiè suì*	12g	Spica Schizonepetae
鲜芦根	*xiān lú gēn*	30g	Rhizoma Phragmitis

[Process of treatment]

Two days after hospitalization, the fever was relieved, body temperature was 36.7℃, the listlessness was improved, cough and dyspnea were alleviated, phlegm was reduced. But there was no appetite. The tongue coating was yellow, white and greasy, indicating there was still heat. Then *jīng jiè suì* (Spica Schizonepetae) was removed from the formula, *zhǐ qiào* (Fructus Aurantii) 12g was added. By the third and fourth day, body temperature became normal, cough and dyspnea were reduced, appetite was improved, the tongue coat was thin, and the pulse was slow. Then *Sāng Jú Yǐn* (Mulberry Leaf and Chrysanthemum Beverage, 桑菊饮) was used with modification. Six days later, the patient was cured.

[Case 2]

Wang, 7 months old, hospitalized on January 8, 1960.

The patient suffered from cough and fever for four days, body temperature was 39.5℃, accompanied by panting and occasional vomiting. The manifestations were body temperature of 39.5℃, 52 breaths per minute, reddish complexion, occasional agitation, somnolence, breathing with the head bent, bluish coloration around the mouth, white coating over the root of the tongue, floating and rapid pulse, heart rate of 132 bpm.

[Diagnosis]

pneumonia.

[Pattern differentiation]

internal and external heat

[Treatment principle]

clear heat to remove toxin and relieve superficial pathogenic factors with acrid and cool herbs.

[Formula]

Má Xìng Shí Gān Tāng (Ephedra, Apricot Kernel, Gypsum and Licorice Decoction), with additions.

[Composition]

Chinese Name	Pin Yin	Amount	Latin Name
麻黄	*má huáng*	3g	Herba Ephedrae
杏仁	*xìng rén*	9g	Semen Armeniacae Amarum
生石膏	*shēng shí gāo*	15g	Gypsum Fbrosum
甘草	*gān cǎo*	6g	Radix Glycyrrhizae
丹皮	*dān pí*	6g	Cortex Moutan Radicis
竹茹	*zhú rú*	12g	Caulis Bambusae in Taeniam
鲜芦根	*xiān lú gēn*	30g	Rhizoma Phragmitis
天花粉	*tiān huā fěn*	9g	Radix Trichosanthis
黄连	*huáng lián*	3g	Rhizoma Coptidis

[Process of treatment]

The next day after hospitalization, there was still fever, but the cough, panting and somnolence were improved, vomiting was reduced, the feces were still dry, the tongue was red with yellow coating, the pulse was slightly floating and rapid. Then the *tiān huā fěn* and *huáng lián* (Rhizoma Coptidis) were removed, and *guā lóu rén* (Semen Trichosanthis, 瓜蒌仁) 9g; *Zǐ Xuě Dān* (Purple Snow Elixir) 1.2g were added. Three to four days after hospitalization, the spiritual condition was improved, the feces could be discharged, but there were still panting and rapid breath with sputum and fever, the tongue was red without coating, the pulse was slightly wiry and rapid. Then *Zǐ Xuě Dān* (Purple Snow Elixir) and *guā lóu rén* (Semen Trichosanthis) were removed, *zhè bèi mǔ* (Bulbus Fritillariae Thunbergii) 6g and *jú hóng* (Exocarpium Citri Rubrum, 橘红) 6g were added. Five to six days later, the fever was relieved, there was slight panting, the breath was hoarse with sputum, the tongue coating was thin and white, and the pulse was slow. These manifestations indicated that the superficial pathogenic factors were gradually relieved and there was still some lingering heat. The herbs then used were *xiān lú gēn* (Rhizoma Phragmitis) 30g; *táo rén* (Semen Persicae) 9g; *xìng rén* (Semen Armeniacae Amarum) 9g; *dōng guā zǐ* (Semen Benincasae, 冬瓜子) 9g; *yǐ rén* (Semen Coicis) 9g; *gān cǎo* (Radix Glycyrrhizae) 6g; *jié gěng* (Radix Platycodi) 9g; *pí pa yè* (Folium Eriobotryae, 枇杷叶) 6g; *chuān bèi mǔ* (Bulbus Fritillariae Cirrhosae) 6g; *jú hóng* (Exocarpium Citri Rubrum) 6g. Seven days later, the tongue became clear, the pulse turned moderate, the spiritual condition and appetite were improved. When the patient left the hospital, I prescribed two doses of *Sāng Jú Yǐn* (Mulberry Leaf and Chrysanthemum Beverage) for him.

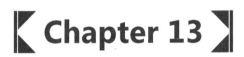

Chapter 13

Treatment of Cough and Dyspnea

Chinese medicine divides cough into different types, such as acute cough, chronic cough, cold cough, heat cough, visceral cough, cough due to qi reversal, cough due to food retention, cough due to lung dryness, lung abscess, lung distension, retention of fluid, invasion of wind and retention of water, etc. Cough was later on divided into two major categories, exogenous cough and endogenous cough.

The lung likes warmth and moisture, and detests cold and dryness. The lung governs the surface of the body and opens into the nose. When exogenous pathogenic factors come into the lung through the nose, it will cause cough. Invisible pathogenic factors, acrid, pungent and dry substance all can directly invade the lung, causing stuffy nose, closure of the pores and inability to sweat. Clinical practice and Chinese medicine theory show that pathogenic cold, heat and water all can cause panting. If the superifical cold is not relieved, it will transform into heat; if sweating cannot be thoroughly induced, it will lead to retention of water below the heart. When confronted with heat, water will be transformed; when confronted with cold, qi will be changed into water. *Má huáng* (Herba Ephedrae) can promote the flow of lung-qi and induce sweating. Therefore, diseases due to lack of sweating can be treated by *má huáng* (Herba Ephedrae). However, in inducing sweating, *má huáng* (Herba Ephedrae) may also cause yang deficiency. With such a condition, the formula for warming yang must be used for supplementation, such as *Má Huáng Fù Zǐ Xì Xīn Tāng* (Ephedra, Aconite and Asarum Decoction). If heat is excessive, water must be insufficient. When the methods for inducing sweating are used, water may also be exhausted. So in using *Yuè Bì Tāng* (Maidservant From Yue Decoction) and *Má Xìng Shí Gān Tāng* (Ephedra, Apricot Kernel, Gypsum and Licorice Decoction), both cold herbs for clearing heat and sweet and cold herbs for nourishing yin should be used to increase the production of fluid.

Panting is either of a deficienct or excess nature. The former is related to the kidney and the latter is related to the lung. The panting caused by invasion of exogenous pathogenic factors is excess in nature while the panting due to endogenous pathogenic factors is deficienct in nature.

The treatment principle is to release stagnant lung-qi. If it is a newly contracted disease, it should be treated by clearing and dissipating therapy; if it is a prolonged disease, it should be treated by warming and transforming therapy. Acute panting and cough are caused by invasion of exogenous pathogenic factors. Chronic panting and cough are due to weakness of the body and should be treated by supporting the healthy qi (*Zhèng qì*).

Wind-cold and Wind-heat Types of Cough and Dyspnea

1. Wind-cold type of panting and cough is a pattern to be treated by *Má Huáng Tāng* (Ephedra Decoction) and is marked by fever, aversion to cold, no sweating, panting, floating and tense pulse, headache, body pain and joint pain. The action of *Má Huáng Tāng* (Ephedra Decoction) is to induce sweating. When sweating is induced, the body will feel warm and aversion to cold and other symptoms will be relieved. If a patient with a cold has no aversion to cold, no body pains, or has a deep and weak pulse, they cannot be treated by *Má Huáng Tāng* (Ephedra Decoction). If the pattern to be treated by *Má Huáng Tāng* (Ephedra Decoction) is accompanied by stiff neck and back, *gé gēn* (Radix Puerariae) can be added.

2. Cough due to Wind-heat or Wind-Warmth disease in the pattern to be treated by *Má Xìng Shí Gān Tāng* (Ephedra, Apricot Kernel, Gypsum and Licorice Decoction) pattern can be treated by *Má Xìng Shí Gān Tāng*

(Ephedra, Apricot Kernel, Gypsum and Licorice Decoction) or *Yuè Bì Jiā Bàn Xià Tāng* (Maidservant From Yue Decoction Plus Pinellia). It is usually treated by formula composed of herbs acrid in taste and cool in nature. But the effect of *Sāng Jú Yǐn* (Mulberry Leaf and Chrysanthemum Beverage) is not as good as that of *Má Xìng Shí Gān Tāng* (Ephedra, Apricot Kernel, Gypsum and Licorice Decoction). Because *má huáng* (Herba Ephedrae) not only induce sweating, but also promote the flow of lung-qi. If *shēng shí gāo* (Gypsum Fbrosum) is used with large dosage, it will be more significant in clearing away heat from the lung and stopping cough. *Má huáng* (Herba Ephedrae) is the key herb for stopping panting. Clinically the use of *má huáng* (Herba Ephedrae) to treat severe panting is sometimes effective for stopping cough, but ineffective for inducing sweating; sometimes effective for promoting urination. Sudden panting due to newly contracted or prolonged diseases, usually marked by high fever, sore-throat, thirst, rapid pulse and acute infectious diseases like pneumonia, can be treated by this formula combined with *Zēng Yè Tāng* (Humor Increasing Decoction, 增液汤) with the addition of *jīn yín huā* (Flos Lonicerae Japonicae), *lián qiào* (Fructus Forsythiae), *bǎn lán gēn* (Radix Isatidis) and *chuān lián* (Rhizoma Coptidis from Sichuan of China, 川连).

Besides, infantile cough is due to invasion of pathogenic heat into the lung and the blood. Prolonged cough will lead to pneumonia or encephal disease with the symptoms of spasmodic cough, reddish complexion, chest stuffiness, sticky sputum difficult to be discharged, dropsy of eyelids, aggravation at night. This disease should be treated immediately by clearing away heat, releasing lung-qi and cooling the blood. The formula is *Má Xìng Shí Gān Tāng* (Ephedra, Apricot Kernel, Gypsum and Licorice Decoction) added with *bái máo gēn* (Rhizoma Imperatae), *shēng dì* (Radix Rehmanniae), *bái sháo* (Radix Paeoniae Alba), *dān pí* (Cortex Moutan Radicis), *bǎi bù* (Radix Stemonae, 百部), *cè bǎi yè* (Cacumen Platycladi, 侧柏叶) and *dǎn nán xīng* (Arisaema cum Bile, 胆南星). If the disease is severe,

Zhì Bǎo Dān (Supreme Jewel Elixir) can be added.

Chronic Cough and Dyspnea

Chronic cough and dyspnea are usually deficient in nature, sometimes complicated by an excess pattern. The treatment of this disease focuses on tonifying deficiency or strengthening the healthy qi (*Zhèng qì*) to eliminate pathogenic factors.

1. Light spasmodic cough, marked by sticky sputum that is difficult to expectorate, upward adverse flow of qi and hoarseness can be treated by *Mài Mén Dōng Tāng* (Radix Ophiopogonis Decoction, 麦门冬汤) combined with *Hòu Pò Xìng Rén Guā Lóu Tāng* (Cortex Magnoliae Officinalis, Semen Armeniacae Amaru and Fructus Trichosanthis Decoction, 厚朴杏仁瓜蒌汤).

2. Cough due to damp phlegm and retention of fluid, accompanied by mild edema, anemia, cold hands and feet, normal urination, no fever, aversion to cold, headache and aching limbs, can be treated by *Xiǎo Qīng Lóng Tāng* (Minor Blue Green Dragon Decoction), and *Líng Gān Wǔ Wèi Jiāng Xīn Tāng* (Poria, Licorice, Fructus Schisandrae, ginger and Asarum Decoction, 苓甘五味姜辛汤).

3. Gastric cough, marked by epigastric focal distention, hypochondriac hardness, constipation and frequent cough can be treated by *Dà Chái Hú Tāng* (Major Bupleurum Decoction, 大柴胡汤), if other medicines cannot help.

4. Cough due to dampness resulting from alcoholism often begins during the change from autumn to winter, and is marked by a spasmodic feeling in the chest, back and flanks as well as an aversion to cold. This can be treated by *Guì Jiāng Cǎo Zǎo Huáng Xīn Fù Tāng* (Cassia Bark, Ginger, Licorice, Jujube, Asarum and Aconite Decoction, 桂姜草枣黄辛附汤).

5. Cough due to spleen and stomach deficiency, *Liù Jūn Zǐ Tāng* (Six

Gentlemen Decoction, 六君子汤) can be used for tonification. In children with a deficient spleen and stomach, who easily contract colds and get coughs that do not stop, can be treated by *Xiǎo Jiàn Zhōng Tāng* (Minor Center Fortifying Decoction) with the addition of other ingredients.

6. Cough due to kidney-dryness and spleen-dampness with the symptoms of diarrhea and poor appetite can be treated by *Hēi Dì Huáng Wán* (Radix Rehmanniae Pill, 黑地黄丸).

7. Non-productive cough due to depressed fire can be treated by *Xiāo Yáo Sǎn* (Free Wanderer Powder, 逍遥散) first and then by *Qīng Zào Jiù Fèi Tāng* (Dryness-Clearing lung-Rescuing Decoction, 清燥救肺汤).

8. Panting, or asthma, can be treated by *Xiǎo Qīng Lóng Tāng* (Minor Blue Green Dragon Decoction). If there is heat, it can be treated by *Xiǎo Qīng Lóng Tāng* (Minor Blue Green Dragon Decoction) combined with *Má Xìng Shí Gān Tāng* (Ephedra, Apricot Kernel, Gypsum and Licorice Decoction). If there are signs of indistinct and thin pulse, aversion to cold and somnolence, *Má Huáng Fù Zǐ Xì Xīn Tāng* (Ephedra, Aconite and Asarum Decoction) can be used with the addition of Hei Xi Dan.

9. Cough in bronchiectasis can be treated by *Qiān Jīn Wěi Jìng Tāng* (Phragmites Stem Decoction), *Xiǎo Xiàn Xiōng Tāng* (Minor Chest Binding Decoction), *Gān Jié Tāng* (Licorice and Platycodon decoction) gand *Tíng Lì Dà Zǎo Xiè Fèi Tāng* (Descurainiae and Jujube lung Draining Decoction, 葶苈大枣泻肺汤).

10. Cough and dyspnea due to cor pulmonale can be treated by *Zhēn Wǔ Tāng* (True Warrior Decoction) combined with *Má Xìng Shí Gān Tāng* (Ephedra, Apricot Kernel, Gypsum and Licorice Decoction) and *Shēn Sū Yǐn* (Ginseng and Perllia Beverage, 参苏饮). If edema is severe, *Xiǎo Shuǐ Shèng Yù Tāng* (Reduce Water to Sagely Cure Decoction) can be added. If there are symptoms of hepatomegaly with ascites, the mixture of *Zhēn Wǔ Tāng* (True Warrior Decoction) and *Yuè Bì Tāng* (Maidservant From Yue Decoction) can be used with the addition of herbs for activating the blood

and promoting urination.

11. Cardiac cough (pulmonary emphysema in modern medicine), marked by chest oppression, shortness of breath, barrel chest, occasional chest pain, and enlarged fingertips can be treated by *Xīn Ké Tāng* (Decoction for Cardiac Cough, 心咳汤) developed by Wang Xu-gao in the Qing Dynasty.

Commonly Used Methods to Treat Cough and Dyspnea Based on Differentiation of Phlegm

1. Cough with yellow phlegm in newly contracted or old disease can be treated by *Má Xìng Shí Gān Tāng* (Ephedra, Apricot Kernel, Gypsum and Licorice Decoction) and *Zēng Yè Tāng* (Humor Increasing Decoction) with the addition of *jīn yín huā* (Flos Lonicerae) and *lián qiào* (Fructus Forsythiae) for clearing heat to remove toxin.

2. Cough with thin phlegm and damp sounds in auscultation can be treated by *Xiǎo Qīng Lóng Tāng* (Minor Blue Green Dragon Decoction). If there is irritability, *shēng shí gāo* (Gypsum Fbrosum) can be added.

3. Cough with thick sputum, gurgling sound in the throat and dry sounds in auscultation can be treated by *Shè Gān Má Huáng Tāng* (Belamcanda and Ephedra Decoction).

4. Cough with with thin and thick sputum and mixed sounds in auscultation can be treated by *Hòu Pò Má Huáng Tāng* (Officinal Magnolia Bark and Ephedra Decoction, 厚朴麻黄汤).

5. Cough with foamy sputum, rapid pulse and palpitations can be treated by *Má Xìng Shí Gān Tāng* (Ephedra, Apricot Kernel, Gypsum

and Licorice Decoction) combined with *Guā Lóu Xiè Bái Bàn Xià Tāng* (Trichosanthes, Chinese Chive and Pinellia Decoction) and *Shēng Mài Sǎn* (Pulse Engendering Powder).

6. Cough with purulent sputum, especially in the morning, with Painful Chest-Obstruction and periodic hematemesis can be treated by *Qiān Jīn Wěi Jìng Tāng* (Phragmites Stem Decoction).

7. Cough in tuberculosis can be treated by *Shēng Mài Sǎn* (Pulse Engendering Powder), *Mài Mén Dōng Tāng* (Radix Ophiopogonis Decoction), *Zhú Yè Shí Gāo Tāng* (Lophatherum and Gypsum Decoction).

8. Cough with profuse sticky sputum that is difficult to expectorate, marked by dyspnea and inability to lie down flat, can be treated by *Zào Jiǎ Wán* (Fructus Gleditsiae Pill) recorded in the Jin Gui (Synopsis of Gold Cabinet).

● Prescription Appendix:

Hēi Dì Huáng Wán (**Radix Rehmanniae Pill**) developed by Liu He-jian (刘河间):

Chinese Name	Pin Yin	Amount	Latin Name
苍术	*cāng zhú*	8g	Rhizoma Atractylodis (soaked in rice water)
熟地黄	*shú dì huáng*	8g	Radix Rehmanniae Praeparata
五味子	*wǔ wèi zǐ*	4g	Fructus Schizandrae
干姜	*gān jiāng*	0.5g	Rhizoma Zingiberis

Hēi Xī Dān (Galenite Elixir, 黑锡丹): Recorded in the book entitled *Tài Píng Huì Mín Hé Jì Jú Fāng* (Imperial Grace Pharmacy Formulas, 太平惠民和剂局方).

Chinese Name	Pin Yin	Latin Name
金铃子	*jīn líng zǐ*	Fructus Toosendan
胡芦巴	*hú lú bā*	Semen Trigonellae
木香	*mù xiāng*	Radix Aucklandiae

Chinese Name	Pin Yin	Latin Name
附子	fù zǐ	Radix Aconiti Lateralis Preparata
肉豆蔻	ròu dòu kòu	Semen Myristicae
补骨脂	bǔ gǔ zhī	Fructus Psoraleae
沉香	chén xiāng	Lignum Aquilariae Resinatum
小茴香	xiǎo huí xiāng	Fructus Foeniculi
阳起石	yáng qǐ shí	Actinolitum
肉桂	ròu guì	Cotex Cinnamomi
黑锡	hēi xī	Galenite
硫黄	liú huáng	Sulfur

Xiǎo Xiàn Xiōng Tāng (Minor Chest Binding Decoction, 小陷胸汤): Developed by Zhang Zhong-jing (张仲景).

Chinese Name	Pin Yin	Latin Name
瓜蒌	guā lóu	Fructus Trichosanthis
川黄连	chuān huáng lián	Rhizoma Coptidis from Sichuan Province of China
半夏	bàn xià	Rhizoma Pinelliae

Shēn Sū Yǐn (Ginseng and Perllia Beverage, 参苏饮): Developed by Tang Rong-chuan (唐容川) , which could treat stagnated blood attacking the lung.

Chinese Name	Pin Yin	Latin Name
人参	rén shēn	Radix Ginseng
苏木	sū mù	Lignum Sappan

Xiǎo Shuǐ Shèng Yù Tāng (Reduce Water to Sagely Cure Decoction, 消水圣愈汤): Developed by Chen Xiu-yuan (陈修园).

Guì Zhī Tāng (Cinnamon Twig Decoction) in the Jin Gui (Synopsis of Gold Cabinet), deleting *sháo yào* (Chinese herbaceoous peony), adding *Má Huáng Xì Xīn Fù Zǐ Tāng* (Herba Ephedrae, Herba Asari and Radix Aconiti Lateralis Preparata Decoction, 麻黄细辛附子汤) as well as *zhī mǔ* (Rhizoma Anemarrhenae).

Xīn Ké Tāng (Decoction for Cardiac Cough, 心咳汤): Developed by Wang Xu-gao (王旭高)

Chinese Name	Pin Yin	Amount	Latin Name
北沙参	běi shā shēn	9g	Radix Glehniae
生石膏	shēng shí gāo	9g	Gypsum Fbrosum
薄荷	bò he	3g	Herba Menthae
牛蒡子	niú bàng zǐ	1.5g	Fructus Arctii
杏仁	xìng rén	9g	Semen Armeniacae Amarum
桔梗	jié gěng	1.5g	Radix Platycodi
甘草	gān cǎo	1.5g	Radix Glycyrrhizae
麦冬	mài dōng	9g	Radix Ophiopogonis
半夏	bàn xià	9g	Rhizoma Pinelliae
茯神	fú shén	9g	Sclerotium Poriae pararadicis
远志	yuǎn zhì	1.5g	Radix Polygalae
小麦	xiǎo mài	15g	Fructus Tritici

If there is profuse phlegm, *chuān bèi mǔ* (Bulbus Fritillariae Cirrhosae) is added; if there is swollen throat, *bàn xià* (Rhizoma Pinelliae) is removed; if there is profuse sweating, *wǔ wèi zǐ* (Fructus Schizandrae) is added.

Comments

The dosage of this formula is light. It can be monitered according to clinical treatment. *Bò he* (Herba Menthae) in the original formula can be changed into *má huáng* (Herba Ephedrae) 3g; *shā shēn* (Radix glehniae) can be changed into *dǎng shēn* (Radix Codonopsis) 30g; the dosage of *shēng shí gāo* (Gypsum Fbrosum) can be doubled; *yuǎn zhì* (Radix Polygalae) can be increased to 12g; *bàn xià* (Rhizoma Pinelliae) can be increased to 12g; *mài dōng* (Radix Ophiopogonis) can be increased to 15g; *fú líng* (Poria) can be increased to 15g; *gān cǎo* (Radix Glycyrrhizae) and *niú bàng zǐ* (Fructus Arctii) can be increased to 9g; *hòu pò* (Cortex Magnoliae Officinalis) 9g can be added.

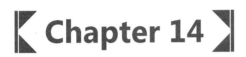

Chapter 14

Treatment of Pleural Diseases

Pleuritis and emphysema are similar to "phlegm disease" and "lung abscess" as recorded in Zhang Zhong-jing's *Jīn Guì Yào Lüè* (Essential Prescriptions of the Golden Coffer). Dampness, rheum, water, and phlegm are all similar, but dampness is formless, while the other three have form. Rheum, water, and phlegm differ in their fluidity. Water is clear, rheum is watery but slightly thicker, while phlegm is sticky and thicker yet.

The following are some of the clinically used therapeutic methods developed according to the symptoms of cold and heat, shortness of breath, pleural effusion, strength of constitution, and duration of the disease.

1. Clearing heat, releasing the exterior, and expelling phlegm: This pattern is characterized by high fever, chest pain, aversion to cold, epigastric focal distention, shortness of breath, slippery or rapid or full pulse, and yellow and greasy tongue coating. Usually *Xiǎo Xiàn Xiōng Tāng* (Minor Chest Binding Decoction) is used together with *Xiǎo Chái Hú Tāng* (Minor Bupleurum Decoction) with the deletion of *gān cǎo* (Radix Glycyrrhizae) and addition of *Yuán huā* (Flos Genkwa, 芫花). If there are symptoms of fever, profuse sputum, vomiting pus-like sticky sputum, cough and shortness of breath, *Qiān Jīn Wěi Jìng Tāng* (Phragmites Stem Decoction) should be added to the formula and the dosage of the herbs for clearing heat to remove toxin should be increased, such as *chuān huáng lián* (Rhizoma Coptidis from Sichuan Province of China), *huáng qín* (Radix Scutellariae), *pú gōng yīng* (Herba Taraxaci) and *Xī Huáng Wán* (Rhinoceros Bezoar Pill, 犀黄丸). If the chest pain is severe, *mǔ lì* (Concha Ostreae) and *jié gěng* (Radix Platycodi) should be added.

2. Draining water: This pattern has chest pain without obvious cold and heat, cough, pleural thickening, wiry pulse and greasy tongue coating. *Mù Fáng Jǐ Tāng* (Radix Stephaniae Tetrandrae Decoction, 木防己汤) recorded in the *Jīn Guì Yào Lüè* (*Essential Prescriptions of the Golden Coffer*) can be used with the addition of *fú líng* (Poria) and *máng xiāo* (Natrii

Sulfas, 芒硝).

3. Warming yang, draining water, transforming qi and harmonizing the middle: This pattern is characterized by cough, shortness of breath, or even inability to lie horizontally, cold limbs, vertigo, weakness, pleural effussion, thin, deep and weak pulse, and light-colored tongue with white coating. *Zhēn Wǔ Tāng* (True Warrior Decoction) and *Yuè Bì Tāng* (Maidservant From Yue Decoction) are used together with modification.

Modifications: For severe chest and hypochondriac pain, *qīng pí* (Pericarpium Citri Reticulatae), *chén pí* (Pericarpium Citri Reticulatae), and *chuān liàn zǐ* (Fructus Toosendan) can be added; for high fever, *Xī Huáng Wán* (Rhinoceros Bezoar Pill) can be added, boiled in water before being taken; for inability to lie horizontally due to cough and dyspnea with thin sputum or vomiting, *Xiǎo Qīng Lóng Tāng* (Minor Blue Green Dragon Decoction) can be used with modification; for distension and pain in the chest and hypochondria without cold and heat, *Mù Fáng Jǐ Tāng* (Radix Stephaniae Tetrandrae Decoction) as recorded in the *Jīn Guì* (Essential Prescriptions of the Golden Coffer) can be used.

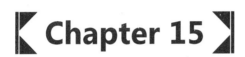

Chapter 15

Treatment of Ulcer Disease

Ulcerative disease is a commonly encountered chronic disease. This disease is usually located in the stomach or duodenum, clinically characterized by regular upper abdominal pain. In Chinese medicine, this disease is called stomach duct pain or heart and abdominal cold pain. There are two main causes of this disease. The first cause is improper eating habits with excessive intake of sweet and greasy foods, over-eating and improper food temperatures. The second cause is stagnation and anger damaging the liver and excessive contemplation and worry damaging the spleen.

● Damage of the stomach by improper food:

Improper food or excessive intake of sweet and greasy foods will lead to dysfunction of the spleen and stomach, resulting in poor appetite, epigastric focal distention and fullness, eructation, acid regurgitation, and hot sensation in the chest. If the stomach cannot get enough nutrients, it will become ulcerated. *Gān Cǎo Xiè Xīn Tāng* (Licorice heart Draining Decoction) can be used to adjust dampness and dryness. The spleen likes warmth and detests aversion to cold. That is why *gān jiāng* (Rhizoma Zingiberis), *wú zhū yú* (Fructus Evodiae), *gāo liáng jiāng* (Rhizoma Alpiniae Officinarum) and *bàn xià* (Rhizoma Pinelliae) are used. The stomach likes to be clear and destests heat. That is why bitter and cold herbs are used to clear heat. This pattern is usually marked by pale tongue, white or yellow greasy tongue coating, and stool that is occasionally dry and occasionally sloppy.

[Formula]

Chinese Name	Pin Yin	Amount	Latin Name
炙甘草	*zhì gān cǎo*	30g	Radix Glycyrrhizae Preparata
党参	*dǎng shēn*	30g	Radix Codonopsis
半夏	*bàn xià*	18g	Rhizoma Pinelliae

Chinese Name	Pin Yin	Amount	Latin Name
川黄连	chuān huáng lián	6g	Rhizoma Coptidis from Sichuan Province of China
干姜	gān jiāng	9g	Rhizoma Zingiberis
高良姜	gāo liáng jiāng	9g	Rhizoma Alpiniae Officinarum
生牡蛎	shēng mǔ lì	18g	Concha Ostreae
乌贼骨	wū zéi gǔ	12g	Os Sepiae (ground)
黄芩	huáng qín	9g	Radix Scutellariae
生姜	shēng jiāng	9g	Rhizoma Zingiberis Recens
大枣	dà zǎo	10 pieces	Fructus Jujubae
延胡索	yán hú suǒ	12g	Rhizoma Corydalis
吴萸	wú yú	9g	Fructus Evodiae

If there is abdominal fullness, add *hòu pò* (Cortex Magnoliae Officinalis) 9g and *jú pí* (Pericarpium Citri Reticulatae) 12g; if there is diarrhea, *chì shí zhī* (Halloysitum Rubrum) 12g and *fú líng* (Poria) 12g can be added; if there is edema, *fú líng* (Poria) 12g and *zé xiè* (Rhizoma Alismatis) 18g can be added.

If the pattern is marked by red tongue, eructation, and heartburn without diarrhea, *Xuán Fù Dài Zhě Tāng* (Flos Inulae and Haematitum Decoction, 旋覆代赭汤) should be used first for several doses, in order to deal with the branch aspect. If there is acid regurgitation, *mǔ lì* (Concha Ostreae) and *wū zéi gǔ* (Os Sepiae) should be added. If there are signs of wiry pulse and liver excess severe pain, *Sì Nì Sǎn* (Frigid Extremities Powder) can be used to harmonize the liver. After taking several doses of these formulas, the patient is treated with *Gān Cǎo Xiè Xīn Tāng* (Licorice heart Draining Decoction) for dealing with the root aspect of the disease.

● Damage of the stomach by emotional excess:

Excessive contemplation and anxiety affect the functions of the spleen and cause ulcerative disease. Liver depression may generate heat, which consumes liver and stomach yin, characterized by insufficiency of gastric liquid and an imbalance between dryness and moistness. Clinically, the manifestations are excessive heat due to yin deficiency and liver excess. The patterns caused are often marked by lack of gastric acid, red or dark-red tongue without coating, dry mouth, wiry pulse, agitation and irritability, dry stool, no acid regurgitation and no heartburn. This is why *Yī Guàn Jiān* (Effective Integration Decoction) is used with the addition of other ingredients for moistening liver-yin and regulating the stomach.

[Formula]

Chinese Name	Pin Yin	Amount	Latin Name
生地	*shēng dì*	18g	Radix Rehmanniae
沙参	*shā shēn*	30g	Radix Adenophorae Strictae
麦冬	*mài dōng*	12g	Radix Ophiopogonis
白芍	*bái sháo*	9g	Radix Paeoniae Alba
枸杞子	*gǒu qǐ zǐ*	12g	Fructus Lycii
川楝子	*chuān liàn zǐ*	12g	Fructus Toosendan
当归	*dāng guī*	9g	Radix Angelicae Sinensis
延胡索	*yán hú suǒ*	12g	Rhizoma Corydalis
甘草	*gān cǎo*	30g	Radix Glycyrrhizae
山茱萸	*shān zhū yú*	12g	Fructus Corni
川黄连	*chuān huáng lián*	3g	Rhizoma Coptidis from Province of China

In the two types of patterns mentioned above, if the disease goes untreated or is treated incorrectly, then a spleen deficiency and blood insufficiency pattern is brought about. The main symptoms are pale tongue, anemia, reduced appetite, pale complexion, weakness, thin and weak pulse. If the gastric acid is insufficient, *Xiǎo Jiàn Zhōng Tāng* (Minor Center Fortifying Decoction) can be used for soothing the liver, strengthening the spleen and nourishing the blood vessels.

[Formula]

Chinese Name	Pin Yin	Amount	Latin Name
炙甘草	zhì gān cǎo	9g	Radix Glycyrrhizae Preparata
桂枝	guì zhī	9g	Ramulus Cinnamomi
白芍	bái sháo	18g	Radix Paeoniae Alba
生姜	shēng jiāng	9g	Rhizoma Zingiberis Recens
大枣	dà zǎo	7 pieces	Fructus Jujubae
饴糖	Yí táng	30g	Saccharum Granorum

The two types of patterns mentioned above are sometimes caused by spleen deficiency and lack of absorption or qi stagnation and blood stasis, which causes bleeding into the stomach. If the disease is acute, the treatment shouls focus on the branch aspect while at the same time considering the root aspect. If the disease is chronic, the treatment should focus on the root aspect. *Huáng Tǔ Tāng* (Yellow Earth Decoction, 黄土汤) can be used.

Bleeding in ulcerative disease means defecation followed by bleeding which due to spleen deficiency and qi deficiency. Failure of the spleen to govern the blood causes bleeding. *Huáng Tǔ Tāng* (Yellow Earth Decoction) can be used with the additioin of *bái zhú* (Rhizoma Atractylodis Macrocephalae) and *fù zǐ* (Radix Aconiti Lateralis Preparata) for promoting qi movement. In addition, *ē jiāo* (Colla Corii Asini), *shēng dì* (Radix Rehmanniae) and *gān cǎo* (Radix Glycyrrhizae) can be used to nourish the blood and enrich yin. In dealing with bleeding, acrid, warm, and dry herbs should not be used. At the same time, *huáng qín* (Radix Scutellariae) can be used to adjust the effect.

[Formula]

Chinese Name	Pin Yin	Amount	Latin Name
炙甘草	zhì gān cǎo	9g	Radix Glycyrrhizae Preparata
熟地	shú dì	60g	prepared Rhizome of Rehmannia
白术	bái zhú	15g	Rhizoma Atractylodis Macrocephalae

Chinese Name	Pin Yin	Amount	Latin Name
炮附子	*páo fù zǐ*	12g	Radix Aconiti Lateralis Preparata
龙眼肉	*lóng yǎn ròu*	30g	Arillus Longan
阿胶	*ē jiāo*	18g	Colla Corii Asini (melted into the decoction)
黄芩	*huáng qín*	9g	Radix Scutellariae
灶心黄土	*zào xīn huáng tǔ*	120g	Terra Flava Usta (decocted first, with the liquid used to decoct the other herbs)

Bleeding in ulcerative disease causes deficiency of both the heart and spleen due to excessive loss of blood. This should be treated by nourishing both the heart and the spleen. Although bleeding from the collaterals may have stopped, the blood is already deficient, accompanied by weakness, pale complexion, weak pulse, palpitations and restless sleep. This can be treated by *Guī Pí Tāng* (spleen Restoring Decoction, 归脾汤) for nourishing both the heart and the spleen, supporting healthy qi (*Zhèng qì*) and controlling the blood.

[Formula]

Chinese Name	Pin Yin	Amount	Latin Name
炙甘草	*zhì gān cǎo*	18g	Radix Glycyrrhizae Preparata
茯苓	*fú líng*	9g	Poria
白术	*bái zhú*	9g	Rhizoma Atractylodis Macrocephalae
党参	*dǎng shēn*	30g	Radix Codonopsis
黄芪	*huáng qí*	30g	Radix Astragali
龙眼肉	*lóng yǎn ròu*	30g	Arillus Longan
当归	*dāng guī*	12g	Radix Angelicae Sinensis
远志	*yuǎn zhì*	9g	Radix Polygalae
炒枣仁	*chǎo zǎo rén*	15g	Semen Jujubae
木香	*mù xiāng*	4g	Radix Aucklandiae
柏子仁	*bǎi zǐ rén*	9g	Semen Platycladi
灶心土	*zào xīn tǔ*	30g	Terra Flava Usta

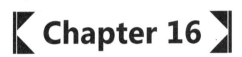

Chapter 16

Treatment of Diarrhea

Diarrhoea is often caused by improper diet, irregular daily activities and invasion of pathogenic factors into the spleen and stomach.

● Diarrhea with indigested food in it (飧泄)

Diarrhea with indigested food in it characterized by aversion to wind, spontaneous sweating, borborygmus, and wiry pulse should be treated by *Wèi Líng Tāng* (stomach Calming Poria Decoction) with the addition of *shēng má* (Rhizoma Cimicifugae) and *fáng fēng* (Radix Saposhnikoviae). Excessive intake of food may damage the intestines and stomach, causing diarrhea with indigested food in it. It should be treated by raising and digestion-promoting therapy. Usually *Mù Xiāng Sǎn* (Radix Aucklandiae Powder, 木香散) can be used. If diarrhea with indigested food in it is marked by wiry pulse, abdominal pain, thirst and slight sweating on the head, it should be treated by *Fáng Fēng Sháo Yào Tāng* (Radix Saposhnikoviae and Chinese Herbaceoous Peony Decoction, 防风芍药汤).

Modified *Mù Xiāng Sǎn* (Radix Aucklandiae Powder):

Mù xiāng (Radix Aucklandiae), *gāo liáng jiāng* (Rhizoma Alpiniae Officinarum), *shēng má* (Rhizoma Cimicifugae), *rén shēn* (Radix Ginseng), *bīng láng* (Semen Arecae), *shén qū* (Massa Medicata Fermentata), *bái zhú* (Rhizoma Atractylodis Macrocephalae), *ròu dòu kòu* (Semen Myristicae), *wú zhū yú* (Fructus Evodiae), *gān jiāng* (Rhizoma Zingiberis), *chén pí* (Pericarpium Citri Reticulatae), *shā rén* (Fructus Amomi).

Fáng Fēng Sháo Yào Tāng (Radix Saposhnikoviae and Chinese herbaceoous peony Decoction):

Fáng fēng (Radix Saposhnikoviae), *bái sháo* (Radix Paeoniae Alba), *huáng qín* (Radix Scutellariae).

● *Táng Xiè* (Sloppy diarrhea, 溏泄)

Sloppy diarrhea is caused by accumulation of turbid substances in the intestines, which is an accumulation of both dampness and heat. It can be treated with *Huáng Qí Sháo Yào Tāng* (Radix Scutellariae and Chinese Herbaceoous Peony Decoction, 黄芪芍药汤) together with *Yì Yuán Săn* (Original Qi Boosting Powder):

Huáng qín (Radix Scutellariae), *bái sháo* (Radix Paeoniae Alba), *gān căo* (Radix Glycyrrhizae), *huá shí* (Talcum) and *zhū shā* (Cinnabaris).

● *Wù Táng* (Duck diarrhea marked by clear urine, dampness and cold, 鹜溏)

This kind of diarrhea is characterized by watery stool, like a duck's, deep and slow pulse, clear and white urine. It can be treated by *Lǐ Zhōng Tāng* (Middle Regulating Decoction) with the addition of *jú hóng* (Exocarpium Citri Rubrum) and *fú líng* (Poria). If the diarrhea cannot be stopped, *fù zǐ* (Radix Aconiti Lateralis Preparata) can be added. Jie-gu said that this kind of diarrhea should be treated by *shēng má* (Rhizoma Cimicifugae), *fù zǐ* (Radix Aconiti Lateralis Preparata), and *gān jiāng* (Rhizoma Zingiberis). Theis decoction should be taken in the morning and evening.

● *Rú Xiè* (Soggy diarrhea, 濡泄)

This kind of diarrhea is marked by heaviness of the body and a soft pulse due to excessive dampness inside the body. Other manifestations are lack of abdominal pain, borborygmus, scanty urine, and watery stool. This can be treated by *Wǔ Líng Săn* (Five Substances Powder with Poria).

● *Huá Xiè* (slippery diarrhea, 滑泄)

This type of diarrhea is chronic and is due to excessive dampness and exhaustion of qi. This should be treated by *Fú Pí Wán* (Supporting spleen Pill, 扶脾丸) or *Bǔ Zhōng Yì Qì Tāng* (Center Supplementing and Qi Boosting Decoction, 补中益气汤) with *hē zǐ* (Fructus Chebulae) and *ròu dòu kòu* (Semen Myristicae) added, or *Sì Zhù Yǐn* (Four Pillar Drink, 四柱饮) or

Liù Zhù Yĭn (Six Pillar Drink, 六柱饮).

Sì Zhù Yĭn is composed of *fú líng* (Poria), *rén shēn* (Radix Ginseng), *fù zĭ* (Radix Aconiti Lateralis Preparata) and *mù xiāng* (Radix Aucklandiae), with the addition of ginger and salt.

Liù Zhù Yĭn is composed of *Sì Zhù Yĭn* with the addition of *ròu dòu kòu* (Semen Myristicae) and *hē zĭ* (Fructus Chebulae).

Fú Pí Wán (Supporting spleen Pill) is composed of *bái zhú* (Rhizoma Atractylodis Macrocephalae), *fú líng* (Poria), *chén pí* (Pericarpium Citri Reticulatae), *hē zĭ* (Fructus Chebulae), *zhì gān căo* (Radix Glycyrrhizae Preparata), *wū méi* (Fructus Mume), *gān jiāng* (Rhizoma Zingiberis), *huò xiāng* (Herba Agastaches), *hóng dòu* (Semen Phaseoli Calcarati, 红豆), *ròu guì* (Cotex Cinnamomi), *mài yá* (Fructus Hordei Germinatus, 麦芽), *shén qù* (Massa Medicata Fermentata) and *hé yè* (Folium Nelumbinis).

● In addition to the above categories, there are other types of diarrhea as listed below:

Stomach diarrhea, marked by yellow complexion and indigestion, which is treated with *Lĭ Zhōng Tāng* (Middle Regulating Decoction).

Spleen diarrhea was marked by vomiting, abdominal distension and violent diarrhea, which is treated with *Xiāng Shā Liù Jūn Zĭ Tāng* (Costusroot and Amomum Six Gentlemen Decoction).

Large intestine diarrhea was marked by urgency to defecate, white colored stool, borborygmus, cutting abdominal pain. This is treated with *Wŭ Líng Săn* (Five Substances Powder with Poria) with the addition of *mù xiāng* (Radix Aucklandiae) .

Small intestine diarrhea, marked by difficult urination, stool with pus and blood, lower abdominal pain. This is treated with *Mù Xiāng Bīng Láng Wán* (Costus Root and Areca Pill, 木香槟榔丸) first and then by *Gĕ Gēn Huáng Qín Huáng Lián Tāng* (Pueraria, Scutellaria, and Coptis Decoction) with the addition of *huá shí* (Talcum).

Kidney diarrhea is marked by diarrhea before dawn and cold abdominal pain. This is treated with *Sì Shén Wán* (Four Spirits Pill, 四神丸) with the addition of *rén shēn* (Radix Ginseng) and *chén xiāng* (Lignum Aquilariae Resinatum); if it is severe, *shú fù zǐ* (Radix Aconiti Lateralis Preparata) and *xiǎo huí xiāng* (Fructus Foeniculi) and *chuān jiāo* (Pericarpium Zanthoxyli) should be used.

Liver diarrhea is marked by abdominal pain and distension due to spleen deficiency and liver excess. This is treated by *Yì Gōng Sǎn* (Special Achievement Powder, 异功散) with the addition of *chuān liàn zǐ* (Fructus Toosendan) and *yuán hú* (Rhizoma Corydalis).

Phlegm diarrhea is marked by fullness in the chest, wiry and slippery pulse. When it is severe, there is vomiting, abdomen feels cold and there is vague pain. This is treated with *Hòu Pò Èr Chén Tāng* (Cortex Magnoliae Officinalis and Two Matured Substances Decoction, 厚朴二陈汤). Obese people tend to have more phlegm. If the pulse is slippery and the patient does not eat but has no sense of hunger, this is phlegm, and *Qīng Zhōu Bái Wán Zǐ* (Qingzhou White Pill, 青州白丸子) can be used to treat the patient.

Food diarrhea is marked by foul-smelling diarrhea, eructation, acid regurgitation, and abdominal pain that is usually alleviated after diarrhea. This is treated with *Xiāng Shā Wèi Líng Tāng* (stomach Calming Poria Decoction) or *Bǎo Hé Wán* (Harmony Preserving Pill, 保和丸) with the addition of *shā rén* (Fructus Amomi) and *ròu dòu kòu* (Fructus Amomi Rotundus).

Da Jia Xie (great mass diarrhea, 大瘕泄) is marked by tenesmus, difficulty to discharge stool, and penis pain. It is due to colddampness transforming into damp-heat. It is diarrhea that is like dysentery but is not dysentery, in which there is the discharge only of watery stool. This is treated with *Bā Zhèng Sǎn* (Eight Corrections Powder) with the addition of *mù xiāng* (Radix Aucklandiae) and *bīng láng* (Semen Arecae).

Alcoholic diarrhea is marked by discharge of stool in the morning due to chronic alcoholism and is treated with *Gě Huā Jiě Chéng Tāng* (Pueraria Flower Liquor-Resolving Decoction, 葛花解醒汤) with the addition of *gé gēn* (Radix Puerariae) and *Xiāng Lián Wán* (Aucklandia and Coptis Pill, 香连丸).

Summer Diarrhea is marked by watery discharge, occurring in the summer, accompanied by a weak and thin pulse, dry mouth, chest oppression and worry. This is due to an attack of summer-dampness. To treat summer diarrhoea, *gé gēn* is the key medicine; to reduce summer fire, *chuān huáng lián* (Rhizoma Coptidis from Sichuan Province of China) should be added; if there is abdominal distension, *hòu pò* (Cortex Magnoliae Officinalis) and *cāng zhú* (Rhizoma Atractylodis) should be added; if there is deficiency, *bái zhú* (Rhizoma Atractylodis Macrocephalae) and *bái biǎn dòu* (Semen Dolichoris, 白扁豆) should be added; if there is food diarrhea in summer, *shén qū* (Massa Medicata Fermentata) and *mù xiāng* (Radix Aucklandiae) should be added; if there is damp diarrhea in summer, *cāng zhú* (Rhizoma Atractylodis), *zé xiè* (Rhizoma Alismatis), *yín huā tàn* (Flos Lonicerae Japonicae Carbonisatum, 银花炭) and *Yì Yuán Sǎn* (Original Qi Boosting Powder) can be added; if there is brown urine, *mù tōng* (Caulis Akebiae, 木通) should be added; if there is vexation, *zhī zǐ* (Fructus Gardeniae) and *dàn zhú yè* (Herba Lophatheri, 淡竹叶) or *huáng qín tàn* (Radix Scutellariae) should be added; if there is vomiting, *bàn xià* (Rhizoma Pinelliae), *hòu pò* (Cortex Magnoliae Officinalis), *zhú rú* (Caulis Bambusae in Taeniam) and *huò xiāng* (Herba Agastaches) should be added; if there is an attack of summer-heat complicated by retention of cold food, *Lián Lǐ Tāng* (Coptis Rectifying Decoction, 连理汤) should be used.

The types of diarrhea, although complicated, are mainly due to an accumulation of dampness that damages the spleen and stomach. Therefore, draining water is the main therapeutic method. If there is scanty urine, then use draining methods. If urination is normal, do not use draining methods. If there is thirst, the methods for draining water and drying the spleen should not be used. If there are symptoms of brown urine, thirst, yellow tongue coating and rapid pulse, it indicates heat, and cold bitter medicinals such as *huáng lián* (Rhizoma Coptidis) and *huáng qín* (Radix Scutellariae) should be used to treat it. If the urine is short but the color has not changed, and the pulse is deficient, then one should nourish and tonify. Because diarrhea naturally tends to damage the fluids, there are frequently the signs of dry mouth, brown and unsmooth urination that is not frequent, and lack of yellow tongue coating. One should not think that this is heat. One should use wind herbs to dry dampness; if the diarrhea is chronic, use raising lifting medicinals, if the diarrhea is slippery, use consolidating and astringing medicinals to stop it; if there is concurrently external wind, then use exterior releasing medicinals; if there is cold, then warm the middle; if there is food stagnation then disperse and depurate; if there is phlegm then transform it; if there is deficiency then tonify; if there is heat then use clearing methods. One should follow the pattern and treat accordingly.

- ## Nine therapeutic methods for treating diarrhea:

1. Bland elimination of dampness: The formula is *Wǔ Líng Sǎn* (Five Substances Powder with Poria) .

2. Raising and lifting: Diarrhea is a pouring downwards. By raising stomach-qi, often diarrhea will stop on its own. One can use *Bǔ Zhōng Yì Qì Tāng* (Center Supplementing and Qi Boosting Decoction) to accomplish this.

3. Clearing and cooling: This means to eliminate heat with bitter and cold medicinals because heat can cause violent diarrhea. The formula to use is *Huáng Qí Sháo Yào Tāng* (Radix Scutellariae and Chinese herbaceoous peony decoction).

4. Dredging and draining: Phlegm congestion, qi stagnation, and food

retention all can cause diarrhea. Dredging is the way to treat this. The formula to use is *Bǎo Hé Wán* (Harmony Preserving Pill) or *Èr Chén Tāng* (Two Matured Substances Decoction, 二陈汤) with the addition of *shén qū* (Massa Medicata Fermentata), *mài yá* (Fructus Hordei Germinatus), *hǎi gé qiào fěn* (Pulvis Concha Meretricis seu Cyclinae), *mù xiāng* (Radix Aucklandiae) and *bīng láng* (Semen Arecae).

5. Relieving and moderating with sweet herbs: Sweet herbs can relieve and moderate the middle jiao in spastic, urgent conditions of diarrhea. The formulas used are *Sì Jūn Zǐ Tāng* (Four Gentlemen Decoction) and *Xiǎo Jiàn Zhōng Tāng* (Minor Center Fortifying Decoction, 小建中汤).

6. Astringing with sour herbs: Sour herbs sour can astringe and stop diarrhea when the qi is scattered. The formula to use is *Wū Méi Wán* (Fructus Mume Pill).

7. Drying the spleen: The cause of diarrhea is dampness resulting from spleen deficiency. The formulas to use are *Píng Wèi Sǎn* (stomach Calming Powder) and *Wèi Líng Tāng* (stomach Calming Poria Decoction).

8. Warming the kidney: The kidney controls urination and defecation. The formula to use is composed of *bǔ gǔ zhī* (Fructus Psoraleae), *ròu dòu kòu* (Semen Myristicae), *xiǎo huí xiāng* (Fructus Foeniculi), and *wǔ wèi zǐ* (Fructus Schizandrae).

9. Astringe and bind: Prolonged diarrhea will make the intestines slippery. In these cases warming and tonifying formulas do not help, and one must use astringing and binding herbs. One should use *Táo Huā Zhōu* (Peach Blossom Porridge, 桃花粥), *chì shí zhī* (Halloysitum Rubrum), *yǔ yú liáng* (Limonitum, 禹余粮), etc.

Diarrhea can also be due to deficiency of kidney-qi resulting from sexual intercourse right after drinking wine and excessive eating. In a kidney deficient person, this causes damp-heat to drain into the kidney and results in chronic diarrhea that does not stop. This can be treated by *Bā Wèi Wán* (Eight Ingredient Pill) with the addition of extra *shān yào*

(Rhizoma Dioscoreae) and *fú líng* (Poria), and reducing the dose of *dì huáng* (Radix Rehmanniae) by half.

The kidney controls urination and defecation. Prolonged diarrhea tends to exhaust the yin and yang of the kidney. It can be treated by herbs like *bǔ gǔ zhī* (Fructus Psoraleae), *ròu dòu kòu* (Semen Myristicae), *xiǎo huí xiāng* (Fructus Foeniculi), and *wǔ wèi zǐ* (Fructus Schizandrae). Although *chén pí* (Pericarpium Citri Reticulatae) and *cāng zhú* (Rhizoma Atractylodis) are used for strengthening the stomach and eliminating dampness, they can be used to deal with the branch aspect; but excessive taking of these herbs can affect the spleen and damage the fluids.

Damp-heat in late summer can also cause diarrhea and can be treated by herbs for eliminating wind, such as *qiāng huó* (Rhizoma et Radix Notopterygii), *fáng fēng* (Radix Saposhnikoviae), *shēng má* (Rhizoma Cimicifugae), *chái hú* (Radix Bupleuri) and *bái zhǐ* (Radix Angelicae Dahuricae).

Diarrhea with poor appetite is due to weakness of the stomach. It can be treated with *rén shēn* (Radix Ginseng) as the main herb, with *bái biǎn dòu* (Semen Dolichoris) and *chén pí* (Pericarpium Citri Reticulatae).

Diarrhea with indigestion can be treated with *suō shā* (Amomi Villosi Semen seu Fructus, 缩砂), *rén shēn* (Radix Ginseng), and *ròu dòu kòu* (Semen Myristicae), etc.

Diarrhea with abdominal pain should be treated by adding *bái sháo* (Radix Paeoniae Alba), *zhì gān cǎo* (Radix Glycyrrhizae Preparata), *fáng fēng* (Radix Saposhnikoviae), and *mù xiāng* (Radix Aucklandiae).

Diarrhea with weakness of qi should be treated by adding *gé gēn*, *rén shēn* (Radix Ginseng), *bái zhú* (Rhizoma Atractylodis Macrocephalae), and *fú líng* (Poria).

Diarrhea with difficult urination should be treated by adding *chē qián zǐ* (Semen Plantaginis) powder and *mù tōng* (Caulis Akebiae). If there is damp-heat in the middle jiao, *zhū líng* (Polyporus) and *zé xiè* (Rhizoma

Alismatis) should be added.

Diarrhea due to retention of meat should be treated by adding *ròu dòu kòu* (Semen Myristicae), *shān zhā* (Fructus Crataegi), and garlic (Bulbus Allii).

Diarrhea due to cold attack should be treated by *Lǐ Zhōng Tāng* (Middle Regulating Decoction) with the addition of *zǐ sū yè* (Folium Perillae).

Diarrhea due to food retention should be treated by adding *lái fú zǐ* (Semen Raphani, 莱菔子) and *shén qū* (Massa Medicata Fermentata).

Diarrhea with damp-phlegm should be treated by adding *bàn xià* (Rhizoma Pinelliae), *bái zhú* (Rhizoma Atractylodis Macrocephalae), and *fú líng* (Poria).

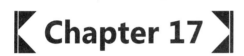

Chapter 17

Treatment of Dysentery

Dysentery is a commonly encounterd infectious disease during the summer. Clinically it can be treated by clearing heat, draining dampness, regulating qi, and resolving stagnation. The most commonly used herbs are *gé gēn* (Radix Puerariae), *huáng qín* (Radix Scutellariae), *huáng lián* (Rhizoma Coptidis), *sháo yào* (Chinese herbaceoous peony), *huá shí* (Talcum), *bīng láng* (Semen Arecae), *hòu pò* (Cortex Magnoliae Officinalis), *guǎng mù xiāng* (Radix Aucklandiae), *fú líng* (Poria), and *jīn yín huā* (Flos Lonicerae).

There is another kind of dysentery, similar to toxic bacillary dysentery in modern medicine, that is acute and changeable, often characterized by simultaneous vomiting and diarrhea, high fever, dehydration, or even unconsciousness. Delayed treatment often causes death. The pathogenesis of dysentery is due to internal retention of damp-heat, food poisoning, and attack by seasonal pathogenic factors. It can be treated by sweating therapy, relieving the superifical pathogenic factors first and then dealing with the internal factors. If heat is not relieved, it will damage the healthy qi (*Zhèng qì*), and worsen the disease.

● Sweating therapeutic methods:

1. Clearing heat to remove toxin first through sweating: The formula used is *Gé Gēn Huáng Qín Huáng Lián Tāng* (Pueraria, Scutellaria, and Coptis Decoction). The dosage for each ingredient is 9-15g, but *gé gēn* (Radix Puerariae) is 30g. *Gé gēn* (Radix Puerariae) is effective at clearing heat to relieve pathogenic factors from the muscles, and therefore is the key herb in the formula. In addition, *má huáng* (Herba Ephedrae) 4.5g; *jié gěng* (Radix Platycodi) 6g; *jīn yín huā* 30g; *bǎn lán gēn* (Radix Isatidis) 15g; *mǎ chǐ xiàn* (Herba Portulacae) 30g; and *Zǐ Xuě Dān* (Purple Snow Elixir) 3g (taken as a draught)should be added to the formula.

2. Resolving stagnation and attacking the internal: This method is used after inducing sweating and removing toxin. About 30 minutes

after taking the previously prescribed formula, the patient is given the second does of the decoction, while at the same time taking *Mù Xiāng Bīng Láng Wán* (Costus Root and Areca Pill), which is composed of *mù xiāng* (Radix Aucklandiae), *bīng láng* (Semen Arecae), *qīng pí* (Pericarpium Citri Reticulatae Viride), *chén pí* (Pericarpium Citri Reticulatae), *é zhú* (Rhizoma Curcumae, 莪术), *huáng lián* (Rhizoma Coptidis), *huáng bǎi* (Cortex Phellodendri), *dà huáng* (Radix et Rhizoma Rhei), *xiāng fù* (Rhizoma Cyperi), and *zhǐ qiào* (Fructus Aurantii). This is taken 2-3 times a day, 9g each time. The decoction is quick in action while the pill is slow in action. That is why the decoction is taken first and the pill second.

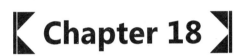

Chapter 18

Treatment of Malaria

Malaria was mentioned early in the *Sù Wèn* (Plain Questions). The location of the disease is in the *shaoyang* and can reach the *taiyin* channels as described in *Shāng Hán Lùn* (On Cold Damage). In the *Shāng Hán Lùn* (On Cold Damage), the pattern in the *taiyang* diseases treated with *Guì Zhī Má Huáng Gé Gēn Tāng* (Decoction composed of half the ingredients of Ramulus Cinnamomi Decoction and half ingredients of Herba Ephedrae Decoction, 桂枝麻黄葛根汤) and the pattern in the *shaoyang* diseases treated with *Chái Hú Tāng* (Bupleurum Decoction) are quite similar to the patterns of malaria. That is why it is said that malaria often involves the *shaoyang* aspect. The *Huáng Dì Nèi Jīng* (Yellow Emperor's Inner Canon) states that malaria is caused by wind. Wind here refers to heat. Doctors of later generations also believed that malaria was caused by phlegm and often involved the *taiyin* aspect. But these understandings made by later generations are just partially correct.

Generally speaking malaria is caused by wind and summer-dampness, which cause malaria when interacting with the *wèi qì* (defensive qi). The *Huáng Dì Nèi Jīng* (Yellow Emperor's Inner Canon) says that "*wèi qì* (defensive qi) descends one section a day". That is why malaria attcks at fixed times. This explanation may not be quite reasonable, but people in ancient times understood that malaria attacked at fixed times, as seen in clinical practice.

Zhang Zhong-jing said: *"The pulse in malaria is wiry. If it is wiry and rapid, there must be heat; if it is wiry and slow, there must be cold; if it is wiry and slow, it can be treated by warming; if it is wiry and tense, it can be treated by sweating through acupuncture and moxibustion; if it is floating and large, it can be treated by vomiting; if it is wiry and rapid, it can be treated by adjusting the diet."*

Zhang's words indicate that wind is the key factor responsible for malaria. That is why a wiry pulse appears in the patterns due to cold or heat or phlegm or retention of food. That is also why it can be treated with warming, purging and vomiting therapeutic methods. Among these methods, sweating is the most important one. If malaria is marked by a normal pulse, no cold, fever, joint pain and vexation, it can be treated by *Bái Hǔ Guì Zhī Tāng* (White Tiger Plus Ramulus Cinnamomi Decoction, 白虎桂枝汤) (in order to inducing sweating). If it is marked by more cold and less heat, it can be treated with *Shǔ Qī Sǎn* (Dichroa Leaf Powder, 蜀漆散); if it is marked by chills and no fever, it can be treated by *Chái Hú Guì Jiāng Tāng* (Bupleurum Cinnamon Ginger Decoction, 柴胡桂姜汤). Malaria nodules can be treated with *Biē Jiǎ Jiān Wán* (Turtle Shell Decocted Pill).

● Treatment based on pattern differentiation

This disease is marked by chills first and then fever, followed by sweating. It attacks regularly. After attack, the patient appears normal. Some cases are characterized by alternating chills and fever. In some patients there is only vomiting. In some children, the manifestation is just convulsions. The basic feature of this disease is an attack at fixed times.

● Treatment:

1. According to the regularity of the disease's attack, the first half of the decoction is taken one hour before the attack and the liquid of the second half of the decoction is taken half an hour before the attack. After taking the medicine, the patient is covered with a blanket in order to induce sweating before the appearance of aversion to cold. Such a treatment is summarized from the idea in the *Shāng Hán Lùn* (On Cold Damage) that *"If fever cannot be relieved after spontaneous sweating, it means disharmony of wèi qì (defensive qi) and can be treated by Guì Zhī Tāng (Cinnamon Twig Decoction)"*.

2. Inducing sweating. If sweating is not induced after taking the medicine, there will be no effect. If it is in winter or autum and if the patient is old, sweating can be induced by covering the patient with a

blanket and soaking the feet in hot water.

3. Regulation. The patient should not eat too much food. During the course of treatment, the patient should stop taking any cold food and avoid washing feet and hands with cold water.

● Essentials for treatment:

1. If there appear symptoms of chills, fever and pain, *Chái Hú Guì Zhī Tāng* (Bupleurum and Cinnamon Twig Decoction, 柴胡桂枝汤) can be used.

2. If there is more fever and less chills, *Guì Zhī Tāng* (Cinnamon Twig Decoction) and *Yuè Bì Tāng* (Maidservant From Yue Decoction) can be used. The ratio of the two types of formulas is 2:1.

3. If the ratio of fever and chills is the same, then *Guì Zhī Má Huáng Gě Gēn Tāng* (Decoction compose of half of the ingredients of Ramulus Cinnamomi Decoction and half ingredients of the Herba Ephedrae Decoction) can be used.

4. If it attacks after overstrain or during pregnancy, it can be treated with *Xiǎo Chái Hú Tāng* (Minor Bupleurum Decoction) with the deletion of *bàn xià* (Rhizoma Pinelliae) and the addition of *tiān huā fěn* (Trichosanthes).

5. Malaria nodule with hypochondriac mass can be treated with *Biē Jiǎ Jiān Wán* (Turtle Shell Decocted Pill).

6. Common formulas: If the symptoms mentioned above are difficult to differentiate, *Dá Yuán Yǐn* (Membrane-Source Opening Beverage, 达原饮), *Cāng Zhú Bái Hǔ Tāng* (White Tiger Decoction Composed of Rhizoma Atractylodis, 苍术白虎汤) and *Xiǎo Chái Hú Tāng* (Minor Bupleurum Decoction) can be used with modification.

General formula developed by the author:

Chinese Name	Pin Yin	Amount	Latin Name
柴胡	*chái hú*	9-15g	Radix Bupleuri
常山	*cháng shān*	3-6g	Radix Dichroae

Chinese Name	Pin Yin	Amount	Latin Name
厚朴	*hòu pò*	9g	Cortex Magnoliae Officinalis
生石膏	*shēng shí gāo*	18g	Gypsum Fbrosum
甘草	*gān cǎo*	9g	Radix Glycyrrhizae
当归	*dāng guī*	9g	Radix Angelicae Sinensis
麻黄	*má huáng*	6g	Herba Ephedrae
葛根	*gé gēn*	9g	Radix Puerariae
苍术	*cāng zhú*	9g	Rhizoma Atractylodis
草果	*cǎo guǒ*	9g	Fructus Tsaoko
生姜	*shēng jiāng*	9g	Rhizoma Zingiberis Recens
大枣	*dà zǎo*	4 pieces	Fructus Jujubae
知母	*zhī mǔ*	12g	Rhizoma Anemarrhenae

7. If the disease is prolonged and tends to recur, *Hé Rén Yǐn* (Flowery Knotweed and Ginseng Beverage, 何人饮) can be used.

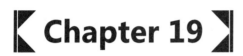

Chapter 19

Treatment of Poliomyelitis

Poliomyelitis is aninfectous disease due to toxin, often occurring in children. It is marked by infection in the respiratory tract, is contagious, and often spreads during the summer and autumn.

Poliomyelitis in Chinese medicine is childhood wind strike in warm disease theory. The early symptoms are sudden fever, vomiting, agitation, somnolence, profuse sweating or no sweating. This is similar to infantile paralysis according to Wang Qing-ren (王清任). According to clinical experience, this disease should be put under the "*Wind strike*" category.

"Wind" in Chinese medicine may refer to the nerve system or sudden attack of disease or climatic change. "*Wind strike*" refers to the symptoms of invasion into the nerve system. Because this is classified as childhood wind strike within the warm diseasetheory, its treatment focuses on clearing heat to remove toxin, regulating the liver, eliminating wind, opening obstruction (Bi) and penetrating the collaterals. The formula used is *Gě Gēn Huáng Qín Huáng Lián Tāng* (Pueraria, Scutellaria, and Coptis Decoction) with the addition of other ingredients. During convalescence, *Jīn Gāng Wán* (Metal Strength Pill) can be used along or with the addition of other ingredients. Clinical practice shows that early treatment ensures better result, and early use of the herbs for clearing heat to remove toxin can shorten convalescence and avoid sequela.

● Treatment principle:

At the acute stage, this disease should be treated by clearing heat to remove pathogenic factors from the surface of the body, eliminating evils with fragrant herbs, regulating the liver, eliminating wind, and penetrating the collaterals. During convalescence, it should be treated by nourishing the liver and kidney, strengthening the tendons and bones, and warming and nourishing the qi and blood.

● Compostion of the formulas:

Gě Gēn Huáng Qín Huáng Lián Tāng (Pueraria, Scutellaria, and Coptis Decoction) with the addition of other ingredients at the acute stage:

Chinese Name	Pin Yin	Amount	Latin Name
生石膏	*shēng shí gāo*	18g	Gypsum Fbrosum
葛根	*gé gēn*	12g	Radix Puerariae
甘草	*gān cǎo*	9g	Radix Glycyrrhizae
金银花	*jīn yín huā*	12g	Flos Lonicerae
杭芍药	*háng sháo yào*	12g	Radix Paeoniae Alba
川黄连	*chuān huáng lián*	4.5g	Rhizoma Coptidis from Sichuan Province of China
黄芩	*huáng qín*	9g	Radix Scutellariae
全蝎	*quán xiē*	3g	Scorpio
蜈蚣	*wú gōng*	3g	Scolopendra

These ingredients are decocted in 600ml of water. *Shí gāo* (Gypsum Fibrosum) is decocted for 15 minutes first and then the other ingredients are put into the pot to decoct. These ingredients are finally decocted into 120-150ml of decoction, to be taken in three doses.

Infantile paralysis is an acute, infectious disease and pertains to the concept of warm disease. The pathogenic factor invades the body through the mouth and nose, entering into the intestines and stomach and causing disease in the *du* vessel. The symptoms often appear in the four limbs, abdominal wall, face and head. At the early stage, the typical symptoms are fever, vomiting and diarrhea, and then followed by flaccid paralysis. Fever is *taiyang* warm disease and should be treated by externally releasing the pathogenic factors. That is why *Yuè Bì Tāng* (Maidservant From Yue Decoction) is used. Vomiting and diarrhea indicate that the disease is located in the intestines and stomach, which is why *Gě Gēn Huáng Qín Huáng Lián Tāng* (Pueraria, Scutellaria, and Coptis Decoction) is used. Since the paralysis originated from the *du* vessel, the dosage of *gé gēn* (Radix Puerariae), *wú gōng* (Scolopendra) and *quán xiē* (Scorpio) is large. To deal with epidemic toxin, *jīn yín huā* (Flos Lonicerae) and *lián qiào* (Fructus Forsythiae) are used for removing toxin. Toxin must be removed, otherwise the healthy qi (*Zhèng qì*) will be damaged. *Sháo yào* (Chinese herbaceoous peony) is used to eliminate blood stagnation; *gān cǎo* (Radix Glycyrrhizae) and the related herbs are used for removing toxin; *má huáng* (Herba Ephedrae) and *gé gēn* (Radix Puerariae) are used to induce sweating. If the patient is treated early and nursed well, the duration of the disease will be shortened, the sequela will be reduced and the course of disease will be restricted to 3-6 months.

● Modifications:

At the early stage, one should use *Zhì Bǎo Dān* (Supreme Jewel Elixir) or *Ān Gōng Niú Huáng Wán* (Peaceful Palace Bovine Bezoar Pill) and *Zǐ Xuě Dān* (Purple Snow Elixir) (if there is diarrhea, *Zǐ Xuě Dān* should not be used). If there is no sweating, *má huáng* (Herba Ephedrae) is added. If there is fever, *dà qīng yè* (Folium Isatidis), *bǎn lán gēn* (Radix Isatidis), and *lián qiào* (Fructus Forsythiae) are added. If there is agitation, *lóng dǎn cǎo* (Radix Gentianae) and *gōu téng* (Ramulus Uncariae Cumuncis) are added. If there is pain, *tiān má* (Rhizoma Gastrodiae) and *sháo yào* (Chinese herbaceoous peony) are added. For penetrating the collaterals, *dì lóng* (Pheretima) and *jiāng cán* (Bombyx Batryticatus) are added. If the paralysis is in the lower limbs, *niú xī* (Radix Achyranthis Bidentatae) and *sāng jì shēng* (Ramus Loranthi) are added. If the paralysis is located in the upper limbs, *chuān xiōng* (Rhizoma Chuanxiong), *dì lóng* (Pheretima) and *sāng jì shēng* (Ramus Loranthi) are added. If there is a distorted face, *xì xīn* (Herba Asari), *xīn yí* (Flos Magnoliae, 辛夷), *chuān xiōng* (Rhizoma Chuanxiong) and *bái zhǐ* (Radix Angelicae Dahuricae) are added. If there are signs of summer-heat, *huò xiāng* (Herba Agastaches) and *huá shí* (Talcum) are added. If there is vomiting, *bàn xià* (Rhizoma Pinelliae), *chén pí* (Pericarpium

Citri Reticulatae) and *zhú rú* (Caulis Bambusae in Taeniam) are added. If there is constipation, *Dà Chái Hú Tāng* (Major Bupleurum Decoction) is used with the additionn of *máng xiāo* (Natrii Sulfas), *chē qián zǐ* (Semen Plantaginis), *dì fū zǐ* (Fructus Kochiae) and *Zǐ Xuě Dān* (Purple Snow Elixir). At the advanced stage, *Jīn Gāng Wán* (Metal Strength Pill) is used with the addition of other ingredients.

During convalescence, the key formula is *Jīn Gāng Wán* (Metal Strength Pill) with the addition of other ingredients:

Chinese Name	Pin Yin	Amount	Latin Name
草薢	*bì xiè*	30g	Rhizoma Dioscoreae Hypoglaucae
杜仲	*dù zhòng*	30g	Cortex Eucommiae
菟丝子	*tù sī zǐ*	15g	Semen Cuscutae
肉苁蓉	*ròu cōng róng*	30g	Herba Cistanches
巴戟天	*bā jǐ tiān*	30g	Radix Morindae Officinalis
天麻	*tiān má*	30g	Rhizoma Gastrodiae
僵蚕	*jiāng cán*	30g	Bombyx Batryticatus
蜈蚣	*wú gōng*	50 pieces	Scolopendra
全蝎	*quán xiē*	30g	Scorpio
木瓜	*mù guā*	30g	Fructus Chaenomelis
牛膝	*niú xī*	30g	Radix Achyranthis Bidentatae
乌贼骨	*wū zéi gǔ*	30g	Os Sepiae
精制马钱子	*jīng zhì mǎ qián zǐ*	60g	Semen Strychni (this must be prepared to remove toxins)

These ingredients are made into honeyed pills of 3g in weight, 1-2 pills each time, 1-3 times a day.

Bì xiè (Rhizoma Dioscoreae Hypoglaucae) is an herb for promoting urination, draining dampness, clearing heat and removing toxin; *dù zhòng* (Cortex Eucommiae) is effective for tranquilization, stopping pain, strengthening bones and tendons, nourishing the liver and the kidney; *tù sī zǐ* (Semen Cuscutae) can moisten the five *zang* organs, nourish the marrow and strengthen the tendons; *bā jǐ tiān* (Radix Morindae Officinalis) can eliminate wind, strengthen tendons, nourish the kidney and enrich the essence. *Tiān má* (Rhizoma Gastrodiae) is added for relieving pain of the four limbs and tendons; *niú xī* (Radix Achyranthis Bidentatae) and *mù guā* (Fructus Chaenomelis) can strengthen the waist, feet and tendons; *jiāng cán* (Bombyx Batryticatus) is effective for eliminating wind and resolving phlegm; *quán xiē* (Scorpio) and *wú gōng* (Scolopendra) are effective for eliminating wind, activating the collaterals and adjusting the nerves. The patient may suffer from weakness of the bones, so *wū zéi gǔ* (Os Sepiae) is added to supplement calcium. *Yín yáng huò* (Herba Epimedii) is effective for warming yang and nourishing the kidney. According to modern medicine, the use of *sāng jì shēng* (Ramus Loranthi) can inhibit the toxin of poliomyelitis; *sāng jì shēng* (Ramus Loranthi) can nourish tendons and bones. This formula is quite effective for eliminating dampness, removing toxin, eliminating wind, penetrating the collaterals, nourishing the liver and the kidney, strengthening the bones and tendons, and exciting the nerves of the spinal cord at the convalescent stage of poliomyelitis.

● Modifications:

After the disappearance of fever and occurrence of paralysis, the formulas used are *Dāng Guī Bǔ Xuè Tāng* (Chinese Angelica blood Supplementing Decoction), *Huáng Qí Guì Zhī Wǔ Wù Tāng* (Astragalus and Cinnamon Twig Five Substances Decoction, 黄芪桂枝五物汤), *Guì Zhī Fù Zǐ Xì Xīn Tāng* (Ramulus Cinnamomi, Radix Aconiti Lateralis Preparata and Herba Asari Decoction, 桂枝附子细辛汤), and *Dāng Guī Sì Nì Tāng* (Chinese Angelica Frigid Extremities Decoction, 当归四逆汤).

● Therapeutic effect:

In 1958, I made the clinical observation of 179 cases of poliomyelitis treated at the Children's Hospital. Among them, 151 were hospitalized right after onset of the disease and 28 were hospitalized half a month to one month after onset of the disease. The following was the result of treatment:

	Full recovery	Basic recovery	Improvement	Total number
Consulation right after illness	77	38	36	151
Consultation half a month or a month after illness	6	3	19	28
Total	83	41	55	179

• Essentials for nuring children with infantile paralysis:

Infantile paralysis is caused by infection of neurotropic toxins. This kind of disease sometimes also affects adults. When one person is infected, the other people around him will also be infected. Sometimes no symptoms appear. Sometimes it can be healed automatically. Fever and vomiting are the typical symptoms of this disease. The patients were usually quite all right in the evening, but the next morning their upper or lower limbs could not move. Delayed or wrong treatment will lead to serious sequela. When this disease has occurred, the patient must be isolated for 40 days.

1. When this disease has occurred, the patient should be helped to lie in a supine position with the legs bent. A pillow is put beneath the popliteal fossa of the patient to fixate the legs.

2. At the early stage, the affected child should rest quietly to rehabilitate the function of the affected limbs. Exercise should not be used too early lest deformity be caused.

3. After the fever is relieved, the muscles should be massged 2-3 times a day, half an hour each time.

4. Hot compresses are applied to the local region to keep the legs warm.

5. Sterilize vomitus.

【 Case Study 】

Cao, male, 6 years old (case number: 164457)

In July 14, 1958, the patient came to the hospital. He had had a fever for three days, accompanied by spurting vomiting, somnolence and listlessness. After hospitalization, a lumbar puncture was performed and was negative. The diagnosis was fever to be examined. On July 15, the following symptoms occurred: paralysis, difficulty swollowing, vomiting foam, constipation, fever of 38℃, somnolence and shortness of breath.

[Physical examination]

the left eye could not be fully closed, the left nasolabial groove became shallow, there was difficulty in talking, the neck was stiff, the knee reflex test was negative, cerebrospinal fluid cells were high, and albumen was negative. Blood test: red blood cell count was 40,000,000/mm^3, hemoglobin 12.2g%; white blood cell count was 6,650/mm^3, lymph 40%, acidophil 2%. A consultation was made that day. The tongue coating was white and thick.

This pattern was due to warm disease wind strike. The treatment should focuse on clearing heat to stop vomiting and resolving turbidity with fragrant herbs. The herbs used were:

Chinese Name	Pin Yin	Amount	Latin Name
鲜藿香	xiān huò xiāng	12g	Fresh Herba Agastaches
薄荷	bò he	9g	Herba Menthae
佩兰	pèi lán	12g	Herba Eupatorii
厚朴	hòu pò	9g	Cortex Magnoliae Officinalis
生石膏	shēng shí gāo	18g	Gypsum Fbrosum
陈皮	chén pí	12g	Pericarpium Citri Reticulatae
竹茹	zhú rú	15g	Caulis Bambusae in Taeniam
川黄连	chuān huáng lián	4.5g	Rhizoma Coptidis from Sichuan Province of China

Continued

Chinese Name	Pin Yin	Amount	Latin Name
蚕砂	*cán shā*	12g	Excrementum Bombycis
姜半夏	*jiāng bàn xià*	12g	Rhizoma Pinelliae Prepared with Ginger
滑石	*huá shí*	12g	Talcum
甘草	*gān cǎo*	9g	Radix Glycyrrhizae

Zhì Bǎo Dān (Supreme Jewel Elixir, 至宝丹) 1 capsule. Since *Zhì Bǎo Dān* (Supreme Jewel Elixir) was difficult to take, lotus root powder was used to dilute the pill into a liquid for oral taking). On July 16, three doses of *Gě Gēn Huáng Qín Huáng Lián Tāng* (Pueraria, Scutellaria, and Coptis Decoction) were prescribed with the addition of other ingredients. On July 17, the patient became conscious, but there was excessive phlegm and drool. After taking six doses of the medicines, the phlegm and drool were reduced. But there were still dry feces, difficulty in swallowing, and a foul smell in the mouth. To deal with such symptoms, the method for clearing the stomach was used. The formula used was *Gě Gēn Huáng Qín Huáng Lián Tāng* (Pueraria, Scutellaria, and Coptis Decoction) with the addition of *huò xiāng* (Herba Agastaches) 9g; *chén pí* (Pericarpium Citri Reticulatae) 12g; *fǎ bàn xià* (Rhizoma Pinelliae Praeparatum) 12g; *jié gěng* (Radix Platycodi) 12g and *gōu téng* (Ramulus Uncariae Cumuncis) 12g. On July 28, the patient's spirit was improved. The previous formula was used with the addition of *shí chāng pú* (Rhizoma Acori Tatarinowii) 9g and *shè gān* (Rhizoma Belamcandae, 射干) 4.5g. At the same time 13 grains of *Liù Shén Wán* (Six Spirits Pill) were used, 4 grains each time. On the afternoon of July 30, the patient could take food and defecate normally.

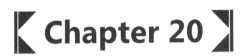

Chapter 20

Treatment of Epilepsy Pattern

● Introduction:

Doctors in the the past divided epilepsy into three categories, wind epilepsy, fright epilespy and food epilepsy.

Wind epilepsy is caused by interior stirring of liver-Wind; food epilepsy is caused by improper diet. In terms of the cause of disease, epilepsy can still be divided into another three categories, phlegm-rheum epilepsy, rheum epilepsy and worm epilepsy.

According to clinical pattern differentiation, wind epilepsy is mainly marked by convulsions accompanied by headache, and should be treated by suppressing yang and eliminating wind. The formula used is *Fēng Yǐn Tāng* (Wind-Eliminating Decoction, 风引汤); food epilepsy is marked by convulsions due to food retention, often seen among children, and should be treated by purgation; phlegm-rhem epilepsy should be treated by resolving phlegm; and rheum epilepsy should be treated by removing fluid retention.

● Treatment:

The following are some of the commonly used therapeutic methods:

1. The common type of epilepsy tends to recur after being treated with phenytoin sodium. This type of epilepsy is marked by convulsions often accompanied by headache and dizziness, and should be treated by suppressing yang, harmonizing the liver, promoting defecation and eliminating phlegm. The commonly used formula is *Chái Hú Lóng Gǔ Mǔ Lì Tāng* (Radix Bupleuri, Os Draconis and Ostrea Decoction) composed of:

Chinese Name	Pin Yin	Amount	Latin Name
柴胡	*chái hú*	18g	Radix Bupleuri
黄芩	*huáng qín*	9g	Radix Scutellariae
半夏	*bàn xià*	12g	Rhizoma Pinelliae
芍药	*sháo yào*	9g	Chinese herbaceoous peony

Chinese Name	Pin Yin	Amount	Latin Name
炙甘草	*zhì gān cǎo*	9g	Radix Glycyrrhizae Preparata
丹参	*dān shēn*	30g	Radix Salviae Miltiorrhizae
桂枝	*guì zhī*	9g	Ramulus Cinnamomi
茯苓	*fú líng*	12g	Poria
生龙骨	*shēng lóng gǔ*	18g	Os Draconis
牡蛎	*mǔ lì*	18g	Concha Ostreae
大黄	*dà huáng*	9g	Radix et Rhizoma Rhei
生姜	*shēng jiāng*	9g	Rhizoma Zingiberis Recens
大枣	*dà zǎo*	10 pieces	Fructus Jujubae

These ingredients are decocted in water. Each dose is decocted twice, to be taken in the morning and evening respectively.

2. Phlegm epilepsy can be treated by *Méng Shí Gǔn Tán Wán* (Chlorite Phlegm Removing Pill, 礞石滚痰丸), 9g in the morning and evening respectively. This formula is used for two days in order to remove phlegm. From the third day on, the commonly used formula, above mentioned, is used.

3. Rheum epilepsy is marked by thin phlegm, shortness of breath and epigastric fullness. This pattern should be treated by transforming rheum and eliminating phlegm. The formula used is *Xiǎo Qīng Lóng Tāng* (Minor Blue Green Dragon Decoction) composed of:

Chinese Name	Pin Yin	Amount	Latin Name
麻黄	*má huáng*	6g	Herba Ephedrae
五味子	*wǔ wèi zǐ*	9g	Fructus Schizandrae
半夏	*bàn xià*	12g	Rhizoma Pinelliae
桂枝	*guì zhī*	9g	Ramulus Cinnamomi
白芍	*bái sháo*	9g	Radix Paeoniae Alba
甘草	*gān cǎo*	9g	Radix Glycyrrhizae
细辛	*xì xīn*	6g	Herba Asari
干姜	*gān jiāng*	9g	Rhizoma Zingiberis

These ingredients are decocted in water. Each dose is decocted twice, to be taken in the morning and evening respectively.

4. Chronic epilepsy may linger for years, maybe with many days between attacks. If there is phlegm or rheum, the treatment should first be based on pattern differentiation above. Because chronic diseases often have deficiency at the root, one should focus on the root treatment with the following formula: *shēng má* (Rhizoma Cimicifugae) 120g; *bèi mǔ* (Bulbus Fritillariae, 贝母) 60g; *tián luó* (Viviparus seu Cipangopaludinae, 田螺) (dryed) 60g; *jì yú* (crucian carp, 鲫鱼) 1 fish, dried, weighing about 60g. These ingredients are ground into a fine powder and made into pills with honey, each weighing 6g; 1 pill taken in the morning and evening. This formula must be used for a long time before it takes effect.

5. Frequently occuring epilepsy often occurs several times each day and is often accompanied by headache and dizziness. It can be treated with modified *Fēng Yǐn Tāng* (Wind-Eliminating Decoction). The ingredients include:

Chinese Name	Pin Yin	Amount	Latin Name
生龙骨	*shēng lóng gǔ*	18g	Os Draconis
生牡蛎	*shēng mǔ lì*	18g	Concha Ostreae
生石膏	*shēng shí gāo*	18g	Gypsum Fbrosum
寒水石	*hán shuǐ shí*	12g	Calcitum
紫石英	*zǐ shí yīng*	30g	Fluoritum
赤石脂	*chì shí zhī*	18g	Halloysitum Rubrum
滑石	*huá shí*	12g	Talcum
干姜	*gān jiāng*	9g	Rhizoma Zingiberis
桂枝	*guì zhī*	9g	Ramulus Cinnamomi
甘草	*gān cǎo*	9g	Radix Glycyrrhizae
大黄	*dà huáng*	6g	Radix et Rhizoma Rhei
地龙	*dì lóng*	12g	Pheretima
全蝎	*quán xiē*	3g	Scorpio

These ingredients are decocted in water twice and taken in two doses. When the symptoms are improved, the common formula is used. After taking the medicines prescribed, the disease recurs once over half a month. When phenytoin sodium is stopped, the disease becomes worsened. Then the formula for treating epilepsy is used.

6. Worm epilepsy is marked by severe headache, white spots over the face, and red spots on the tip of the tongue. *Rén Shēn Bài Dú Yǐn* (Ginseng Toxin-Vanquishing Beverage, 人参败毒饮) is used with the addition of *xióng huáng* (Realgar), *Wū Méi Wán* (Fructus Mume Pill) 30g, or *Huà Chóng Wán* (Worm-Transforming Pill, 化虫丸).

Huà Chóng Wán (Worm-Transforming Pill):

Chinese Name	Pin Yin	Amount	Latin Name
雄黄	*xióng huáng*	30g	Realgar
雷丸	*léi wán*	60g	Omphalia
干漆	*gān qī*	30g	Resina Toxicodendri
百部	*bǎi bù*	90g	Radix Stemonae
鹤虱	*hè shī*	60g	Fructus Carpesii
枯矾	*kū fán*	30g	Alumen dehydratum
槟榔	*bīng láng*	60g	Semen Arecae
苦楝根皮	*kǔ liàn gēn pí*	30g	Cortex Meliae
川椒	*chuān jiāo*	30g	Pericarpium Zanthoxyli
乌梅	*wū méi*	60g	Fructus Mume

● Note:

These ingredients are made into small pills with water, 6g each time and taken three times a day.

Chái Hú Lóng Gǔ Mǔ Lì Tāng (Radix Bupleuri, Os Draconis and Ostrea Decoction) is the common formula. It can be used with the addition of other ingredients. *Chái hú* (Radix Bupleuri), *lóng gǔ* (Os Draconis) and *mǔ lì* (Concha Ostreae) can harmonize the liver, suppress yang and eliminate wind, applicable to wind epilepsy. *Dān shēn* (Radix Salviae Miltiorrhizae), *lóng gǔ* (Os Draconis) and *mǔ lì* (Concha Ostreae) can nourish the blood and stop convulsion. *Dà huáng* (Radix et Rhizoma Rhei), *gān cǎo* (Radix Glycyrrhizae) and *bàn xià* (Rhizoma Pinelliae) can promote digestion and treat food epilepsy.

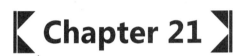

【 Chapter 21 】

Treatment of Trigeminal Neuralgia

Trigeminal neuralgia generally manifests as an acute, paroxysmal painful condition, that is sometimes painful and sometimes not. The cause is still unclear. Generally, analgesics are used or nerve block techniques. If the pain is severe, then the nerves are surgically cut, which can relieve pain, but leads to certain side effects.

Trigeminal neuralgia is known as *Piān Tóu Tòng* (literally meaning wind attacking half of the head, 偏头痛) in Chinese medicine. The clear yang of the six *fu* organs and the Jing-essence of the five *zang* organs all converge at the head. Wind invades the body through the channels. Pathogenic factors produced inside the body, such as stagnation of qi, blood or phlegm, can cause obstruction, which will also lead to pain. Half-head pain is related to the *jueyin*, *shaoyang* and *yangming* channels. Dry-heat in the stomach and intestines, wind-fire in the liver and gallbladder, and stagnation of pathogenic factors in these three channels will make the vessels full, swollen and distended, eventually pressing the nerves and causing sudden pain. That is why it attacks and stops intermittently. *Shí gāo* (Gypsum Fibrosum), *huáng qín* (Radix Scutellariae), and *gé gēn* (Radix Puerariae) are used to clear heat from the *yangming* channel. *Chái hú* (Radix Bupleuri) and *huáng qín* (Radix Scutellariae) are used to clear heat from the liver and the gallbladder. *Jīng jiè* (Herba Schizonepetae), *gōu téng* (Ramulus Uncariae Cumuncis), *bò he* (Herba Menthae), *cāng ěr zǐ* (Fructus Xanthii), and *màn jīng zǐ* (Fructus Viticis) are used to expel wind and dissipate fire. *Quán xiē* (Scorpio) and *wú gōng* (Scolopendra) are used to relieve spasm. *Chì sháo* (Radix Paeoniae Rubra) and *gān cǎo* (Radix Glycyrrhizae) are used for activating the blood and subduing swelling.

Composition of the formula:

Chinese Name	Pin Yin	Amount	Latin Name
生石膏	*shēng shí gāo*	24g	Gypsum Fbrosum
葛根	*gé gēn*	18g	Radix Puerariae

Chinese Name	Pin Yin	Amount	Latin Name
黄芩	huáng qín	9g	Radix Scutellariae
赤芍	chì sháo	12g	Radix Paeoniae Rubra
荆芥穗	jīng jiè suì	9g	Herba Schizonepetae
钩藤	gōu téng	12g	Ramulus Uncariae Cumuncis
薄荷	bò he	9g	Herba Menthae
甘草	gān cǎo	9g	Radix Glycyrrhizae
苍耳子	cāng ěr zǐ	12g	Fructus Xanthii
全蝎	quán xiē	6g	Scorpio
蜈蚣	wú gōng	3 pieces	Scolopendra
柴胡	chái hú	12g	Radix Bupleuri
蔓荆子	màn jīng zǐ	12g	Fructus Viticis

If the eyes are painful, *sāng yè* (Folium Mori, 桑叶) and *jú huā* (Flos Chrysanthemi) are added. If toothache is severe, *xì xīn* (Herba Asari), *shēng dì* (Radix Rehmanniae) and *niú xī* (Radix Achyranthis Bidentatae) are added.

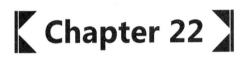

Chapter 22

Treatment of *Bǎi Hé* (Lily Disease)

Bǎi Hé (lily disease) disease also corresponds to *"restless organ disease"* and *"women with feeling of cooked meat stuck in the throat disease"* in Chinese medicine. Usually *Bàn Xià Hòu Pò Tāng* (Pinellia and Officinal Magnolia Bark Decoction) is used to treat this disease, such as *Gān Mài Dà Zǎo Tāng* (Licorice, Wheat and Jujube Decoction). According to the *Jīn Guì Yào Lüè* (*Essential Prescriptions of the Golden Coffer*), *Bǎi Hé* (lily disease) disease means "the disease that is caused by simultaneous involvement of one hundred vessels, marked by desire to eat but difficulty to eat, silence, desire to lie down but difficulty in lying down, desire to walk but difficulty walking, appearance of heat but without heat and appearance of cold but actually not cold, bitter taste in the mouth and brown urine. No herbs can be used to treat it. When the patient has taken medicine, she will violently vomit and have diarrhea."

This disease is greatly related to emotional changes or lingering pathogenic factors in the channels after illness. Bitter taste in the mouth and brown urine indicate that there is heat; dizziness during urination indicates deficiency in the lower part of the body and excess in the upper part of the body. *Bǎi Hé Zhī Mǔ Tāng* (Bulbus Lilii and Rhizoma Anemarrhenae Decoction) can treat the pattern of dizziness during urination.

The existence of pathogenic factors show that this disease is excess in nature, alothough onset after illness indicates deficiency. This disease is characterized by a mixture of deficiency and excess, so it cannot be simply treated by tonifying or purging. In the *Jīn Guì Yào Lüè* (*Essential Prescriptions of the Golden Coffer*), *bǎi hé* (Bulbus Lilii) is the key herb used to treat this disease, since it can treat pathogenic qi, abdominal distention, and heart pain, as well as gently disinhibit urination and the bowels while at the same time tonifying the Middle and benefiting the qi. Because this herb can tonify the healthy qi while not helping the pathogen and attack the pathogen while not harming the healthy qi, it fits this pattern perfectly.

Bàn Xià Hòu Pò Tāng (Pinellia and Officinal Magnolia Bark Decoction) treats the feeling that there is cooked meat stuck in the throat, but it can also be used for chest oppression, epigastric knotted feeling, dry heaves, and a feeling that one cannot swollow down. This is similar to hysteria in modern medicine. Someone with these complaints generally has other signs of depression as well.

In the *Jīn Guì Yào Lüè* (Essential Prescriptions of the Golden Coffer), *Gān Mài Dà Zǎo Tāng* (Licorice, Wheat and Jujube Decoction) is also used to treat hysteria. This formula is only composed of three herbs, which are all quite ordinary in action. Therefore it can treat *Bǎi Hé* (lily disease).

[Case 1]

Li, female, was carried to the hospital because it was difficult for her to walk. She said that she suffered from Painful Chest-Obstruction with the symptoms of chest oppression, palpitations, shortness of breath and dizziness. *Guā Lóu Xiè Bái Bàn Xià Tāng* (Trichosanthes, Chinese Chive and Pinellia Decoction) was prescribed, but it did not work. Careful examination found that the patient had other symptoms, such as depression, desire to cry, eructation and sighing. Then *bǎi hé* (Bulbus Lilii), *dì huáng* (Radix Rehmanniae), *xuán fù huā* (Flos Inulae) and *dài zhě shí* (Haematitum) were added to the formula. After taking the medicine, all the symptoms disappeared.

[Case 2]

Sun, male, said that he was afraid of cold and would put on a fur-lined jacket even in the summer. He suffered from chest oppression, stomachache and abdominal distension. He came to the hospital in autumn, but he had already put on a cotton hat, fur-lined jacket and cotton-padded shoes. The formula prescribed was composed of:

Chinese Name	Pin Yin	Amount	Latin Name
紫苏叶	zǐ sū yè	12g	Folium Perillae
半夏	bàn xià	12g	Rhizoma Pinelliae
厚朴	hòu pò	9g	Cortex Magnoliae Officinalis
生姜	shēng jiāng	9g	Rhizoma Zingiberis Recens
旋覆花	xuán fù huā	12g	Flos Inulae
代赭石	dài zhě shí	15g	Haematitum
陈皮	chén pí	9g	Pericarpium Citri Reticulatae
百合	bǎi hé	30g	Bulbus Lilii
知母	zhī mǔ	12g	Rhizoma Anemarrhenae
生地	shēng dì	12g	Radix Rehmanniae

One month after taking the medicines prescribed, he changed winter clothes into autumn clothes. He said that he was no longer afraid of cold, just felt heat rushing up the diaphragm and chest when he was anxious. He also felt bitter taste in the mouth. The previous formula was used again with the herbs of *Xiǎo Xiàn Xiōng Tāng* (Minor Chest Binding Decoction) added:

Chinese Name	Pin Yin	Amount	Latin Name
旋覆花	xuán fù huā	12g	Flos Inulae
代赭石	dài zhě shí	18g	Haematitum
滑石	huá shí	12g	Talcum
苏叶	sū yè	12g	Folium Perillae
知母	zhī mǔ	12g	Rhizoma Anemarrhenae
百合	bǎi hé	30g	Bulbus Lilii
厚朴	hòu pò	9g	Cortex Magnoliae Officinalis
半夏	bàn xià	12g	Rhizoma Pinelliae
生甘草	shēng gān cǎo	9g	Radix Glycyrrhizae
川黄连	chuān huáng lián	6g	Rhizoma Coptidis from Sichuan Province of China
蚕砂	cán shā	15g	Excrementum Bombycis
栝蒌	guā lóu	30g	Fructus Trichosanthis

He was eventually cured.

[Case 3]

Zhao, female, frequently cryed and laughed with the symptoms of sweating, palpitations and neurosis.

The formrula prescribed contained:

Chinese Name	Pin Yin	Amount	Latin Name
五味子	wǔ wèi zǐ	12g	Fructus Schizandrae
沙参	shā shēn	30g	Radix Adenophorae Strictae
麦冬	mài dōng	12g	Radix Ophiopogonis
炙甘草	zhì gān cǎo	9g	Radix Glycyrrhizae Preparata
小麦	xiǎo mài	30g	Fructus Tritici
大枣	dà zǎo	10 peices	Fructus Jujubae
知母	zhī mǔ	12g	Rhizoma Anemarrhenae
百合	bǎi hé	30g	Bulbus Lilii
云苓	yún líng	15g	Poria from Yunnan Province of China

After taking sixteen doses of the formula, most of the symptoms were alleviated significantly, but she felt feverish on her palms and soles, and the sweating was not improved. The herbs prescribed were:

Chinese Name	Pin Yin	Amount	Latin Name
生甘草	shēng gān cǎo	9g	Radix Glycyrrhizae
丹皮	dān pí	12g	Cortex Moutan Radicis
沙参	shā shēn	30g	Radix Adenophorae Strictae
地骨皮	dì gǔ pí	12g	Cortex Lycii
小麦	xiǎo mài	30g	Fructus Tritici
大枣	dà zǎo	10 pieces	Fructus Jujubae
知母	zhī mǔ	12g	Rhizoma Anemarrhenae
百合	bǎi hé	30g	Bulbus Lilii
生地	shēng dì	12g	Radix Rehmanniae

After taking eight doses, the feverish sensation over the palms and soles disappeared, but the urine was yellow and there was a burning sensation during urination. The herbs prescribed were:

Chinese Name	Pin Yin	Amount	Latin Name
五味子	*wǔ wèi zǐ*	9g	Fructus Schizandrae
麦冬	*mài dōng*	12g	Radix Ophiopogonis
沙参	*shā shēn*	30g	Radix Adenophorae Strictae
知母	*zhī mǔ*	12g	Rhizoma Anemarrhenae
百合	*bǎi hé*	30g	Bulbus Lilii
生地	*shēng dì*	12g	Radix Rehmanniae
生甘草	*shēng gān cǎo*	9g	Radix Glycyrrhizae
小麦	*xiǎo mài*	30g	Fructus Tritici
大枣	*dà zǎo*	10 pieces	Fructus Jujubae
滑石	*huá shí*	12g	Talcum

After taking 8 doses, she was cured.

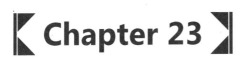

Chapter 23

Treatment of Neurasthenia

Neurasthenia pertains to the concepts of *"deficiency-taxation"*, *"insomnia"*, *"palpitations"*, *"kidney deficiency"* and *"non-interaction between the heart and kidney"* in Chinese medicine. People in ancient times divided this disease into two kinds: damage of the Ying-nutritive and damage from the emotions.

Damage from the emotions means damage of the five *zang* organs. Although any of the five *zang* organs may be damaged in this disease, the main one to be damaged is the heart, the next is the spleen, the kidney, the liver and the lung. The heart stores the Shen-Spirit, while the spleen is damaged by worry, the liver by anger, the kidney by fear, and the lung by sorrow.

The main symptoms of this disease are insomnia, palpitations, shortness of breath, dizziness, headache, low back ache, weakness in the legs, and poor memory. The following are the clinically treated types:

● Deficiency of both the heart and spleen:

This type is characterized by insomnia, palpitations, shortness of breath, frequent sighing, poor appetite, thin and white tongue coating, thin and weak pulse. This pattern should be treated by nourishing both the heart and the spleen. The formula used is *Guī Pí Wán* (spleen Restoring Pill, 归脾丸) and *Bǔ Xīn Dān* (heart Supplementing Elixir, 补心丹).

● Kidney deficiency:

This type is usually seen among males, characterized by dizziness, poor memory, poor concentration and dreaminess. It can be treated by *Qǐ Jú Dì Huáng Wán* (Lycium Berry, Chrysanthemum and Rehmannia Pill) together with *Guì Zhī Lóng Gǔ Mǔ Lì Tāng* (Cinnamon Twig, Os Draconis and Ostrea Decoction).

1. Kidney-yin deficiency: This type is characterized by low back ache, weakness in the legs, dizziness that is relatively severe; there may be

headache, nocturnal seminal emissions, red tongue, yellow tongue coating or no coating, thin and rapid pulse, weak pulse at the Chi (Cubit-proximal) position, especially on the left hand. The treatment should be focused on nourishing yin and calming the mind. The formula used is *Qǐ Jú Dì Huáng Wán* (Lycium Berry, Chrysanthemum and Rehmannia Pill) together with *Zhū Shā Ān Shén Wán* (Cinnabar Spirit Calming Pill).

2. Excessive kidney-fire due to yin deficiency: This type is characterized by frequent nocturnal seminal emissions, spermatorrhea, yellow urine, no tongue coating, or red tongue with yellow coating, thin and rapid pulse. This should be treated by nourishing the yin to reduce fire. The formula used is *Zhī Bǎi Dì Huáng Wán* (Anemarrhena, Phellodendron and Rehmannia Pill, 知柏地黄丸), with modification, or *Dà Bǔ Yīn Wán* (Major Yin Supplementing Pill, 大补阴丸).

3. Kidney-yang deficiency: This type is characterized by low back ache, weakness in the legs, and aversion to cold; there may be impotence and premature ejaculation. The treatment should be focused on enriching the source of fire and eliminating turbidity. The formula used is *Jīn Guì Shèn Qì Wán* (Golden Coffer Kedney Qi Pill).

● Anxiety due to deficiency of heart-yang:

This type is characterized by anxiety and insomnia due to overstrain. The treatment should be focused on nourishing the blood, harmonizing the liver and calming the mind. The formula used is *Suān Zǎo Rén Tāng* (Sour Jujube Decoction, 酸枣仁汤) or *Sì Wù Ān Shén Tāng* (Four Substances for Spirit Calming Decoction, 四物安神汤).

● Deficiency of heart-yin and predominance of heart-Fire:

This type is characterized by agitation, red tongue, rapid pulse and dry mouth. The formula used is *Huáng Qín Huáng Lián Ē Jiāo Jī Zǐ Huáng Tāng* (Radix Scutellariae, Rhizoma Coptidis, Colla Corii Asini and Vitellus

Galli Decoction).

● Blood deficiency and damage of the fluids:

In this pattern, the blood and fluids of the heart, liver, and kidney is damaged, which gives rise to fire that harasses upwards and causes insomnia with excessive dreams, agitation, palpitations, dry mouth, red or dry tongue, thin and rapid pulse. The treatment should focus on nourishing the blood and calming the mind. The formulas used are *Bŭ Xīn Dān* (heart Supplementing Elixir) and *Zhū Shā Ān Shén Wán* (Cinnabar Spirit Calming Pill).

● Phlegm-dampness disturbing the stomach:

This type is characterized by discomfort of the stomach, nausea, vomiting, no desire to drink water, insomnia, white and greasy tongue coating, and a moderate pulse. The treatment should be focused on regulating the stomach, eliminating phlegm and calming the mind. The formula used is *Wēn Dǎn Tāng* (gallbladder Warming Decoction) with the addition of other ingredients or *Bàn Xià Shú Mǐ Tāng* (Pinellia and Broomcorn Millet Decoction, 半夏秫米汤).

When this disease is chronicit can be difficult to cure, and generally takes quite a long time. That is why pills are usually used. Acute cases are easier and quicker to change. The treatment should be prompt and stronger. Therefore, decoctions are used.

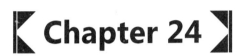

Chapter 24

Treatment of Wind Stroke

Wind patterns are usually located in the liver. Although it is called *"wind stroke"*, this disease involves the *du* vessel, and is not caused by pathogenic wind. Liu He-jian says, "Most wind diseases are in fact caused by severe heat. This heat transforms into wind-dryness, but heat is the most important factor." It is necessary to differentiate deficiency and excess as well as cold and heat in dealing with wind stroke.

Clinically, three points are very important in diagnosing wind stroke: numbness of the fingers, perceptual disturbances of local areas in the limbs, subjective feeling of sudden mental confusion. Those who are over 40 years old must be very careful if such phenomena have appeared in the last year or two.

During the unconsciousness/coma stage, treatment can be given by blowing a little *Tōng Guān Sǎn* (Gate-Freeing Powder, 通关散) into the nose. This formula is composed of *xì xīn* (Herba Asari), *fǎ bàn xià* (Rhizoma Pinelliae Praeparatum) and *zào jiǎ* (Fructus Gleditsiae), which are ground into a fine powder. Such a treatment is helpful for resuscitating the patient. If the patient sneezes, the prognosis is favorable; if the patient does not sneeze, the prognosis is unfavorable. Then the juice of *shēng jiāng* (Rhizoma Zingiberis Recens) and *bái fán* (Alumen) is poured into the mouth of the patient in order to induce vomiting.

The second step is to take *Zài Zào Wán* (Re-creation Pill, 再造丸) twice a day for 1-2 days. The action of this medicine is to adjust the functions of the nerves, nourish the blood, resolve stagnation, open the collaterals, eliminate wind and adjust the central nervous system. During this period, *Xù Mìng Tāng* (Rescuing life Decoction, 续命汤) also can be used.

The third step is to use *Ān Gōng Niú Huáng Wán* (Peaceful Palace Bovine Bezoar Pill) or *Sū Hé Xiāng Wán* (Storax Pill, 苏合香丸). If there is excess phlegm with heat signs, *Ān Gōng Niú Huáng Wán* (Peaceful Palace Bovine Bezoar Pill) or *Zhì Bǎo Dān* (Supreme Jewel Elixir) can be used. If there is excess heat in *yangming* channel with dry feces and tongue, *Zǐ Xuě*

Dān (Purple Snow Elixir) can be used; if there is dampness, *Sū Hé Xiāng Wán* (Storax Pill) can be used.

These formulas are used till the patient becomes conscious. The treatment of sequela is described in the following:

Paralysis accompanied by high blood pressure can be treated by suppressing yang and opening the collaterals. The formula used is *Fēng Yǐn Tāng* (Wind-Eliminating Decoction), composed of *dà huáng* (Radix et Rhizoma Rhei), *gān jiāng* (Rhizoma Zingiberis), *lóng gǔ* (Os Draconis), *guì zhī* (Ramulus Cinnamomi), *gān cǎo* (Radix Glycyrrhizae), *mǔ lì* (Concha Ostreae), *hán shuǐ shí* (Calcitum), *huá shí* (Talcum), *chì shí zhī* (Halloysitum Rubrum), *bái shí zhī* (Halloysitum Album, 白石脂), *zǐ shí yīng* (Fluoritum), and *shí gāo* (Gypsum Fibrosum). Besides *cí shí* (Magnetitum, 磁石), *guī bǎn* (Plastrum Testudinis, 龟板), *biē jiǎ* (Carapax Trionycis) and *shēng tiě luò* (Frusta Ferri, 生铁落) can be added to the formula. Hyperactivity of yang due to excessive phlegm and high blood pressure can be treated by *Tiān Má Gōu Téng Yǐn* (Gastrodia and Uncaria Beverage) combined with *Lù Yàn Xù Mìng Tāng* (Proved Rescuing life Decoction, 录验续命汤), composed of *má huáng* (Herba Ephedrae), *guì zhī* (Ramulus Cinnamomi), *dāng guī* (Radix Angelicae Sinensis), *rén shēn* (Radix Ginseng), *shí gāo* (Gypsum Fibrosum), *gān jiāng* (Rhizoma Zingiberis), *gān cǎo* (Radix Glycyrrhizae), *chuān xiōng* (Rhizoma Chuanxiong) and *xìng rén* (Semen Armeniacae Amarum). Dry feces, dry tongue and stomach-heat can be treated by *Sān Huà Tāng* (Three Transformations Decoction, 三化汤) or *Tiáo Wèi Chéng Qì Tāng* (stomach Regulating and Purgative Decoction, 调胃承气汤). Paralysis can be treated by *Hóu Shì Hēi Sǎn* (Hou's Black Powder, 侯氏黑散), composed of *jú huā* (Flos Chrysanthemi), *bái zhú* (Rhizoma Atractylodis Macrocephalae), *xì xīn* (Herba Asari), *yún líng* (Poria from Yunnan Province of China), *mǔ lì* (Concha Ostreae), *jié gěng* (Radix Platycodi), *fáng fēng* (Radix Saposhnikoviae), *rén shēn* (Radix Ginseng), *bái fán* (Alumen), *huáng qín* (Radix Scutellariae), *dāng guī* (Radix Angelicae Sinensis), *gān jiāng* (Rhizoma Zingiberis), *chuān xiōng* (Rhizoma Chuanxiong) and *guì zhī* (Ramulus Cinnamomi). This decoction should be taken when cooled. If there are no dry feces and no heat, the blood pressure and hypertension are already improved, the sequela are just numbness, weakness, inability to extend limbs and incapability of raising the arm, and it can be treated by strengthening the tendons and bones, opening the channels and activating the collaterals. The formula used is *Guì Zhī Tāng* (Cinnamon Twig Decoction) with the addition of *huáng qí* (Radix Astragali), *dāng guī* (Radix Angelicae Sinensis), *dù zhòng* (Cortex Eucommiae), *xù duàn* (Radix Dipsaci), *tiān má* (Rhizoma Gastrodiae), *dōng chóng xià cǎo* (Cordyceps), *yín yáng huò* (Herba Epimedii), *jī xuè téng* (Caulis Spatholobi), *xiāng fù* (Rhizoma Cyperi), *wū yào* (Radix Linderae), *gāo liáng jiāng* (Rhizoma Alpiniae Officinarum), *shēn jīn cǎo* (Herba Lycopodii), and *shān zhā* (Fructus Crataegi), etc. When the disease is cured, *Hóu Shì Hēi Sǎn* (Hou's Black Powder) can still be used together with *Liù Wèi Dì Huáng Wán* (Six Ingredient Rehmannia Pill) to consolidate the curative effect.

If there is aphasia, it can be treated by *Zī Shòu Jiě Yǔ Tāng* (Life-Prolonging Speech-Returning Decoction, 资寿解语汤), *Dì Huáng Yǐn Zǐ* (Rehmannia Drink), *Hé Jiān Líng Jiǎo Sǎn* (He-jian's Cornu Saigae Tataricae Powder, 河间羚角散).

Zī Shòu Jiě Yǔ Tāng (Life-Prolonging Speech-Returning Decoction) is composed of:

Chinese Name	Pin Yin	Latin Name
防风	*fáng fēng*	Radix Saposhnikoviae
附子	*fù zǐ*	Radix Aconiti Lateralis Preparata
天麻	*tiān má*	Rhizoma Gastrodiae
酸枣仁	*suān zǎo rén*	Semen Jujubae
羚羊角	*líng yáng jiǎo*	Cornu Gazellae
官桂	*guān guì*	Cortex Cinnamomi
羌活	*qiāng huó*	Rhizoma et Radix Notopterygii
甘草	*gān cǎo*	Radix Glycyrrhizae

Dì Huáng Yǐn Zǐ (Rehmannia Drink) is composed of:

Chinese Name	Pin Yin	Latin Name
熟地	*shú dì*	Prepared Rhizome of Rehmannia
巴戟天	*bā jǐ tiān*	Radix Morindae Officinalis
山萸肉	*shān yú ròu*	Fructus Corni
石斛	*shí hú*	Herba Dendrobii
肉苁蓉	*ròu cōng róng*	Herba Cistanches
附子	*fù zǐ*	Radix Aconiti Lateralis Preparata
五味子	*wǔ wèi zǐ*	Fructus Schizandrae
官桂	*guān guì*	Cortex Cinnamomi
白茯苓	*bái fú líng*	Poria
麦门冬	*mài mén dōng*	Radix Ophiopogonis
石菖蒲	*shí chāng pú*	Rhizoma Acori Tatarinowii
远志	*yuǎn zhì*	Radix Polygalae

Cerebral thrombosis can be treated by activating the blood to resolve stasis. The formula used is *Sì Wù Tāng* (Four Substances Decoction, 四物汤).

Encephalomalacia can be treated by *Bǔ Yáng Huán Wǔ Tāng* (Yang Supplementing and Five Returning Decoction, 补阳还五汤) developed by Wang Qing-ren in the Qing Dynasty.

The herbs for dealing with wind problems all can be used to treat this disease. Hot herbs can be used, as long as they fit the disease pattern. Herbs in this category that can be used are *fù zǐ* (Radix Aconiti Lateralis Preparata), *gān jiāng* (Rhizoma Zingiberis) and *ròu guì* (Cotex Cinnamomi), etc. The herbs for removing dampness, such as *fú líng* (Poria) and *bái zhú* (Rhizoma Atractylodis Macrocephalae), can be used to promote absorption. Sedatives, such as *lóng gǔ* (Os Draconis), *mǔ lì* (Concha Ostreae), *zǐ shí yīng* (Fluoritum) and *tiě luò* (Frusta Ferri), can be used to lower blood pressure, because in Chinese medicine these herbs are used to "descend counterflow". Herbs for cooling the blood can be used to stop bleeding, and blood moving herbs are used to activate the blood and open the collaterals.

《 Chapter 25 》

Experience in Using *Dì Huáng Yǐn Zǐ* (Rehmannia Drink)

Dì Huáng Yǐn Zǐ (Rehmannia Drink, 地黄饮子) was developed by Liu He-jian (刘河间) for treating disablement, which is a kind of wind stroke. Doctors in ancient times believed that wind stroke involved either the channels, the collaterals, the *fu* organs or the *zang* organs. When it is in *fu* organs, it is usually in the *yangming*. When it is in the *zang* organs, it is usually in the Shao yin-kidney. Wind stroke in Chinese medicine often covers the symptoms of a cerebrovascular accident and facial palsy in modern medicine. During convalescence from cerebral hemorrhage, the treatment is focused on the kidney. Wind stroke with the symptoms of stiff tongue, flaccidity of limbs, choking when taking in food and slow reaction time can be treated by *Dì Huáng Yǐn Zǐ* (Rehmannia Drink).

● Comments on *Dì Huáng Yǐn Zǐ* (Rehmannia Drink)

Dì Huáng Yǐn Zǐ (Rehmannia Drink, 地黄饮子) is based on *Jīn Guì Shèn Qì Wán* (Golden Coffer Kedney Qi Pill), and uses the idea that to treat above, one should treat below.

If there appear symptoms of imbalance between the heart and kidney, knotted and intermittent pulse as well as palpitations, it can be treated with *Guā Lóu Xiè Bái Bái Jiǔ Tāng* (Trichosanthes, Chinese Chive and White Wine Decoction), and *Dāng Guī Sháo Yào Sǎn* (Chinese Angelica and Peony Powder). If there is panting due to failure of the kidney to receive qi, *chén xiāng* (Lignum Aquilariae Resinatum) and *ròu guì* (Cotex Cinnamomi) should be added to warm the kidney. If the kidney does not warm the spleen, spleen-Yang will decline and cause abdominal distension, hiccups and lack of appetite. To treat such a problem, *dǎng shēn* (Radix Codonopsis), *bàn xià* (Rhizoma Pinelliae), *gān jiāng* (Rhizoma Zingiberis), *dīng xiāng* (Flos Caryophylli, 丁香) and *shì dì* (Calyx Kaki, 柿蒂) should be added to warm the spleen. If there appear symptoms of chest oppression and phlegm, *Juān Yǐn Liù Shén Tāng* (Eliminating Rheum Six Spirits Decoction, 蠲饮六神汤) should be used to eliminate phlegm, open the collaterals, regulate qi, harmonize the stomach, relieve stagnation and calm the mind.

[Case 1]

Sun, male, 64 years old, first visit on August 27, 1975.

After an attack of wind stroke, he began to suffer from inflexibility of the right lower limb, difficulty walking, heaviness of the legs, vertigo and headache, slurred speech, choking when eating. He had a wiry pulse that was weak at the Chi (proximal) positions. The disease was located in the liver and kidney.

[Formula]

Chinese Name	Pin Yin	Amount	Latin Name
生地	*shēng dì*	12g	unprepared Rhizome of Rehmannia
熟地	*shú dì*	12g	prepared Rhizome of Rehmannia
牡丹皮	*mǔ dān pí*	12g	Cortex Moutan Radicis
山药	*shān yào*	12g	Rhizoma Dioscoreae
山茱萸	*shān yú ròu*	12g	Fructus Corni
茯苓	*fú líng*	12g	Poria
泽泻	*zé xiè*	12g	Rhizoma Alismatis
肉苁蓉	*ròu cōng róng*	18g	Herba Cistanches
巴戟天	*bā jǐ tiān*	15g	Radix Morindae Officinalis
杜仲	*dù zhòng*	12g	Cortex Eucommiae
黄芪	*huáng qí*	30g	Radix Astragali
当归	*dāng guī*	12g	Radix Angelicae Sinensis
天麻	*tiān má*	12g	Rhizoma Gastrodiae

Second visit was on September 24. After taking several doses of the medicines prescribed, the choking when eating food stopped, but the other symptoms remained unchanged. The previous formula was prescribed again with the addition of *gé gēn* (Radix Puerariae) 18g; *lǜ dòu yī* (Testa Glycinis) 18g; And *zé xiè* (Rhizoma Alismatis) was increased to 30g.

Third visit was on October 11. After taking ten doses of the medicines prescribed, his speech was significantly improved, but the other symptoms remained unchanged. *Dì Huáng Yǐn Zǐ* (Rehmannia Drink) was prescribed with modification.

[Formula]

Chinese Name	Pin Yin	Amount	Latin Name
熟地	*shú dì*	24g	prepared Rhizome of Rehmannia
石斛	*shí hú*	12g	Herba Dendrobii
山萸肉	*shān yú ròu*	12g	Fructus Corni
肉苁蓉	*ròu cōng róng*	18g	Herba Cistanches
麦冬	*mài dōng*	15g	Radix Ophiopogonis
茯苓	*fú líng*	12g	Poria
石菖蒲	*shí chāng pú*	9g	Rhizoma Acori Tatarinowii
五味子	*wǔ wèi zǐ*	9g	Fructus Schizandrae
巴戟天	*bā jǐ tiān*	15g	Radix Morindae Officinalis
天麻	*tiān má*	12g	Rhizoma Gastrodiae
杜仲	*dù zhòng*	12g	Cortex Eucommiae
黄芪	*huáng qí*	30g	Radix Astragali
泽泻	*zé xiè*	30g	Rhizoma Alismatis
稻豆衣	*lǔ dòu yī*	18g	Testa Glycinis

Fourth visit was on January 2. His speech was improved, but he still had headaches. His legs were heavy. The previous formula was prescribed again, but *zé xiè* (Rhizoma Alismatis) and *lǔ dòu yī* (Testa Glycinis) were removed, and *guì zhī* (Ramulus Cinnamomi) 9g was added.

Fifth visit was on Feburary 10. After taking ten doses of the medicines prescribed, his speech became clear, but his voice was low and his legs were still weak. His pulse was wiry and strong, but weak at the Chi regions. *Dì Huáng Yǐn Zǐ* (Rehmannia Drink) was prescribed again with the addition of *dù zhòng* (Cortex Eucommiae) 12g; *tiān má* (Rhizoma Gastrodiae) 12g; *jī xuè téng* (Caulis Spatholobi) 30g. The dosage of *ròu guì*

(Cotex Cinnamomi) and *fù zǐ* (Radix Aconiti Lateralis Preparata) was 6g each.

Sixth visit was on April 27. All of the symptoms were improved. The present manifestations were wiry pulse, weak at the Chi regions, and weakness of the legs. This is kidney deficiency, and lack of nourishment of the sinews. The previous formula was prescribed with the addition of *yín yáng huò* (Herba Epimedii) 30g, and *dōng chóng xià cǎo* (Cordyceps) 9g. The patient took ten doses of the medicines, followed by long-term taking of honeyed pills. On follow-up made one year later, it was found that his illness was cured. The only remaining problem was slow response.

[Case 2]

Gong, male, 77 years old

He suffered from coronary heart disease with atrial fibrillation and hypertension. He was treated in a hospital for one month. After being discharged from that hospital, he was still troubled by cerebral thrombosis, paralysis of the left side of the body, and infection of the lungs. Three weeks later his illness became critical and was treated by modern medicine. At the same time, I was invited for a consultation. The clinical manifestations were blackish complexion, unclear speech, stiff tongue, mental fatigue, excessive sputum, hiccup, choking when eating food, cold sweating, knotted and intermittent pulse, and paralysis of the left side of the body. *Dì Huáng Yǐn Zǐ* (Rehmannia Drink) was used, with the addition of other ingredients according to the conditon of the patient. It began to take effect seven months later. At first, *Dì Huáng Yǐn Zǐ* (Rehmannia Drink) was used with the addition of *xī yáng shēn* (Radix Panacis Quinquefolii, 西洋参) and *huáng qí* (Radix Astragali), because the healthy qi was damaged. When there was hiccup, *Xuán Fù Dài Zhě Tāng* (Flos Inulae and Haematitum Decoction) and *shì dì* (Calyx Kaki) was added. When there was heart failure, *Guā Lóu Xiè Bái Bái Jiǔ Tāng*

(Trichosanthes, Chinese Chive and White Wine Decoction) was used as a supplementary therapy. When there were fever, excessive sputum and unconsciousness, *Zhì Bǎo Dān* (Supreme Jewel Elixir), *shé dǎn* (Fel Serpentis, 蛇胆) and *chén pí* (Pericarpium Citri Reticulatae) were added. After treatment with both Chinese medicine and Western medicine, the patient had a clear consciousness, normal speech, normal swallowing of food, flexible limbs and normal blood pressure. After being discharged from the hospital, the patient's tongue coating disappeared for sometime and his appetite was poor, then *Juān Yǐn Liù Shén Tāng* (Eliminating Rheum Six Spirits Decoction) was prescribed. The follow-up survey made one year later found no abnormal changes.

[Case 3]

Tan, male, over 70 years old.

His symptoms were flaccidity of legs, panting due to phlegm, deafness, stiff tongue and amnesia. *Bàn Xià Hòu Pò Tāng* (Pinellia and Officinal Magnolia Bark Decoction), *Má Xìng Shí Gān Tāng* (Ephedra, Apricot Kernel, Gypsum and Licorice Decoction), and *Wēn Dǎn Tāng* (Gallbladder Warming Decoction) were used first for removing phlegm. Then *Dì Huáng Yǐn Zǐ* (Rehmannia Drink) was used with modification for half a year. The decoction was taken for 30 doses. Then pills were used, with the addition of *lù jiǎo jiāo* (Colla Cornus Cervi) and *dōng chóng xià cǎo* (Cordyceps). After half a year of treatment, all the symptoms were relieved.

[Case 4]

Fan, male, 64 years old.

His symptoms were atrophy of the legs, instability in walking, and heaviness of the head. *Dì Huáng Yǐn Zǐ* (Rehmannia Drink) was used with modification. After taking over 100 doses of the medicines, he was cured.

Explanation of *Dì Huáng Yǐn Zǐ* (Rehmannia Drink)

Dì huáng (**Radix Rehmanniae**) is used to treat damage of the middle, expel blood Bi pattern, enrich marrow, promote the growth of muscles, tonify the five *zang* organs, nourish yin, suppress yang, promote blood production and cool the blood, improve blood deficiency, eliminate taxation heat, eliminate atrophy and palpitations.

In dealing with patterns with knotted and intermittent pulse and palpitations to be treated by *Zhì Gān Cǎo Tāng* (Honey-Fried Licorice Decoction), the dosage of *dì huáng* (Radix Rehmanniae) can be 48g.

Bā jǐ tiān (**Radix Morindae Officinalis**) is effective for expelling pathogenic wind, treating impotence and pain involving the lower abdomen and external genitals, strengthening the tendons and bones, calming the five *zang* organs, supplementing the middle and invigorating qi. Clinical practice has proved that it is quite effective for nourishing the liver and the kidney.

Shí hú (**herba Dendrobii**) is effective for regulating yin and yang, balancing the upper and the lower, nourishing yin and enriching essence, improving deficiency, eliminating blockage and descending qi. It can be used to treat emaciation and tonify the five *zang* organs.

Ròu cōng róng (**Herba Cistanches**) is used to treat five kinds of overstrain and seven kinds of damage by supplementing the middle, strengthening yin and replenishing essence.

Shān yú ròu (**Fructus Corni**) can tonify the liver, eliminate Cold and Heat, remove Damp Bi-Pattern, strengthen yin, stop sweating, can reach all nine orifices and nourish the five *zang* organs.

Wǔ wèi zǐ (**Fructus Schizandrae**) can preserve the essence of the five *zang* organs and six Fu-Organs in the kidney.

Ròu guì (**Cotex Cinnamomi**) is a herb that is yang in nature and that enters the blood-Aspect. It is mainly used for regulating nutrient qi and defensive qi, opening yang, disinhibiting water, descending qi, eliminating stagnation, supplementing the middle, relieving pain and vexation, regulating the pores and interstices, and enhancing the effect of other herbs.

Fú líng (**Poria**) can transform water qi, opens the chest, regulates visceral qi and eliminates dampness. Its main action is to smooth the water pathways and spread water to all parts of the body. It is also used to promote urination, moisten dry mouth and tongue, relieves epigatric pain, stops palpitations, vexation, and cough.

Mài dōng (**Radix Ophiopogonis**) is mainly used to treat shortness of breath, emaciation, impairment of the middle and mass in the chest and abdomen due to damage of stomach-yin and exhaustion of the stomach collaterals. *Mài dōng* (Radix Ophiopogonis) is used to invigorate stomach-yin. In *Zhì Gān Cǎo Tāng* (Honey-Fried Licorice Decoction) developed by Zhang Zhong-jing, *mài dōng* (Radix Ophiopogonis) is used to treat yin deficiency, unsmoothness of the vessels and exhaustion of blood in the vessels. This shows that *mài dōng* (Radix Ophiopogonis) is effective for nourishing yin essence of the stomach, moistening the heart and the lung, as well as dredging the vessels.

Fù zǐ (**Radix Aconiti Lateralis Preparata**) is used to guide qi and activatae yang, and is effective for treating wind-cold disease, atrophy disorder, cough due to adverse flow of qi, spasm, knee pain, abdominal mass, stiff spine and hiccups.

Shí chāng pú (**Rhizoma Acori Tatarinowii**) is used to harmonize, diffuse, and open the mind and tonify the five *zang* organs, dredge the nine orifices, disinhibit the limbs, as well as treat cold-damp Bi-Pattern, cough due to adverse flow of qi, deafness, forgetfulness, and loss of voice.

Yuǎn zhì (**Radix Polygalae**) is used to balance the heart and the kidney, promote kidney-qi to flow to the heart, improve vision and hearing and open the nine orifices.

The discussion of *Dì Huáng Yǐn Zǐ* (Rehmannia Drink) shows that it is an effective dredging and tonifying formula.

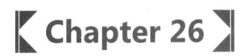

Chapter 26

Treatment of Cold Hernia

Cold hernia was recorded in the *Jīn Guì Yào Lüè* (Essential Prescriptions of the Golden Coffer). Hernia here refers to lower abdominal spasm with protruding mass due to cold. That is why it is called cold hernia.

Cold hernia starts from the kidney and liver channels. It is caused by liver cold that leads to kidney cold. So this disease starts from the liver but appears in the kidney. The liver governs the tendons and the channel and collaterals of the liver run around the lower abdomen and the external genitals. That is why it causes lower abdominal pain. Cold causes spasm. That is why hernia is marked by the symptoms lower abdominal pain and hardness, straight extension of the legs, taut tendons, cold sweating, cold limbs, thin and white tongue coating, and wiry and tense pulse. The treatment should be focused on warming the channels to disperse cold. The formula to be used is *Wū Tóu Guì Zhī Tāng* (Radix Aconiti and Ramulus Cinnamomi Decoction).

[Formula]

Chinese Name	Pin Yin	Amount	Latin Name
桂枝	*guì zhī*	12g	Ramulus Cinnamomi
芍药	*sháo yào*	12g	Chinese herbaceoous peony
甘草	*gān cǎo*	9g	Radix Glycyrrhizae
生姜	*shēng jiāng*	12g	Rhizoma Zingiberis Recens
大枣	*dà zǎo*	10 pieces	Fructus Jujubae
乌头	*wū tóu*	24g	Radix Aconiti
白蜜	*bái mì*	60g	White honey

[Decoction]

Wū tóu (Radix Aconiti) is decocted with honey first. When the liquid has reduced by half, the dregs are removed. *Guì Zhī Tāng* (Cinnamon Twig Decoction) is decocted separately. The two decoctions are mixed together and taken in two doses.

[Cautions]

1. The dosage of formula needs to be large enough to cure the disease. A lower dosage will not work.

2. If the patient appears drunk after taking the medicines prescribed, the effect will be better.

If *Wū Tóu Guì Zhī Tāng* (Radix Aconiti and Ramulus Cinnamomi Decoction) is effective at first and ineffective later on, it is due to blood deficiency because of prolonged illness. If the pulse is wiry and thin, *Dāng Guī Shēng Jiāng yáng Ròu Tāng* (Radix Angelicae Sinensis, Rhizoma Zingiberis Recens and Mutton Decoction) can be used.

[Formula]

Dāng guī (Radix Angelicae Sinensis) 60g; *shēng jiāng* (Rhizoma Zingiberis Recens) 15g; mutton 500g, *chén pí* (Pericarpium Citri Reticulatae) 12g.

[Decoction]

The mutton is decocted in 1500ml of water for some time. Then the mutton is taken out. The *dāng guī* (Radix Angelicae Sinensis), *shēng jiāng* (Rhizoma Zingiberis Recens) and *chén pí* (Pericarpium Citri Reticulatae) are put into the mutton decoction to decoct into 400ml. The decoction is taken in the morning and evening.

This decoction will take effect immediately if *Wū Tóu Guì Zhī Tāng* (Radix Aconiti and Ramulus Cinnamomi Decoction) is ineffective.

If the patient has a concurrent qi-level disease, which in the *Jīn Guì Yào Lüè* is described as a hard disk the size of a plate below the heart, it can be treated by *Guì Zhī Tāng* (Cinnamon Twig Decoction) with the deletion of *sháo yào* (Chinese herbaceoous peony) and the addition of *Má Huáng Xì Xīn Fù Zǐ Tāng* (Herba Ephedrae, Herba Asari and Radix Aconiti Lateralis

Preparata Decoction).

[Formula]

Chinese Name	Pin Yin	Amount	Latin Name
桂枝	guì zhī	9g	Ramulus Cinnamomi
生姜	shēng jiāng	9g	Rhizoma Zingiberis Recens
甘草	gān cǎo	9g	Radix Glycyrrhizae
大枣	dà zǎo	6 pieces	Fructus Jujubae
麻黄	má huáng	9g	Herba Ephedrae
附子	fù zǐ	9g	Radix Aconiti Lateralis Preparata
细辛	xì xīn	6g	Herba Asari

Case comments

Years ago I treated a man named Han, 50 years old, who had suffered from cold hernia for two years. He went to Henan and Shandong to receive treatment, but there was no effect. The manifestations were thin and white tongue coating, wiry and thin pulse, lower abdominal pain and hardness, stiffness of legs, cold limbs and cold sweating. *Wū Tóu Guì Zhī Tāng* (Radix Aconiti and Ramulus Cinnamomi Decoction) was prescribed and one dose proved to be effective. After taking 20-30 doses, he was still not fully cured. Then *Dāng Guī Shēng Jiāng Yáng Ròu Tāng* (Radix Angelicae Sinensis, Rhizoma Zingiberis Recens and Mutton Decoction) was used and the patient was eventually cured.

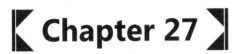

【 Chapter 27 】

Treatment of Male Sterility

Male sterility is caused either by immature sperm or by impotence. The person with immature sperms may be normal in the other viscera. It is not caused by other diseases, but by weakness of the body. The nature of this disease is cold essence. Cold means that the essence is insufficient. *Tiān Xióng Sǎn* (Tianxiong Aconite Powder, 天雄散) can be used to deal with this disease.

Male sterility is located in the kidney, but it is also related to the spleen, liver and heart. In *Tiān Xióng Sǎn* (Tianxiong Aconite Powder), *bái zhú* (Rhizoma Atractylodis Macrocephalae) is used in large dosage. The treatment principle is tonifying both the kidney and the spleen, warming yang and replenishing essence. In this formula, *fù zǐ* (Radix Aconiti Lateralis Preparata) and *guì zhī* (Ramulus Cinnamomi) are used for warming yang; *bái zhú* (Rhizoma Atractylodis Macrocephalae) is used for strengthening the spleen; and *shēng lóng gǔ* (Os Draconis) is used for suppressing yang and nourishing yin. *Tiān Xióng Sǎn* (Tianxiong Aconite Powder) is recorded in *Jīn Guì Yào Lüè* (*Essential Prescriptions of the Golden Coffer*). In ancient times, loss of semen was divided into two kinds: one was seminal emission without dreaming; the other was seminal emission with dreaming. The former is due to deficiency complicated by cold and can be treated by *Tiān Xióng Sǎn*; the latter is due to damage of heart-Spirit and can be treated by *Guì Zhī Tāng* (Cinnamon Twig Decoction). Use *lóng gǔ* (Os Draconis) and *mǔ lì* (Concha Ostreae) to astringe essence. The term "loss of essence" which was used in ancient times means speratorrhea in modern times. *Tiān Xióng Sǎn* (Tianxiong Aconite Powder) is now often used with the addition of other ingredients, such as *ròu cōng róng* (Herba Cistanches), *gǒu qǐ* (Fructus Lycii), *bā jǐ tiān* (Radix Morindae Officinalis), *yín yáng huò* (Herba Epimedii), *dōng chóng xià cǎo* (Cordyceps), *dǎng shēn* (Radix Codonopsis) and *dāng guī* (Radix Angelicae Sinensis) for replenishing essence, supplementing marrow, invigorating qi and nourishing the blood. During treatment, the patient should avoid sexual intercourse.

【 Case Study 】

Sun, male, married for 4 years without child.

His semen was 16,000,000-21,000,000/ml, the activity was about 30%-50%. Methyltestosterone did not help. The manifestations were dizziness, fatigue, lumbago, aversion to cold, impotence, premature ejaculation, deep and thin pulse that was weak at the Chi positions, and white tongue coating. This was insufficiency of kidney-yang. Methods for warming yang, replenishing essence and invigorating qi were used.

[Formula]

Chinese Name	Pin Yin	Amount	Latin Name
附子	fù zǐ	12g	Radix Aconiti Lateralis Preparata
白术	bái zhú	18g	Rhizoma Atractylodis Macrocephalae
肉桂	ròu guì	6g	Cotex Cinnamomi
生龙骨	shēng lóng gǔ	18g	Os Draconis
牡蛎	mǔ lì	18g	Concha Ostreae
韭菜子	jiǔ cài zǐ	15g	Semen Allii Tuberosi
当归	dāng guī	12g	Radix Angelicae Sinensis
肉苁蓉	ròu cōng róng	18g	Herba Cistanches
枸杞子	gǒu qǐ zǐ	9g	Fructus Lycii
巴戟天	bā jǐ tiān	12g	Radix Morindae Officinalis
党参	dǎng shēn	30g	Radix Codonopsis
淫羊藿	yín yáng huò	18g	Herba Epimedii
冬虫夏草	dōng chóng xià cǎo	6g	Cordyceps

After taking 30 doses of the medicines prescribes, his premature ejaculation was cured and other symptoms were improved. His wife was pregnant soon thereafter.

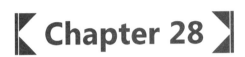

Chapter 28

Treatment of Lupus Erythematosus

Lupus erythematosus is a modern medical disease name. It is similar to the diseases of "*Lì Fēng*" (Pestilence Wind, 疠风) and "*Ròu Jí*" (Extreme of the Flesh, 肉极) in Chinese medicine. According to the theory of Chinese medicine, the treatment of this disease should be focused on adjusting the nutrient-qi (*yíng qì*) and the defensive qi (*wèi qì*), while at the same time adjusting the body's healthy qi and clearing the toxin. Differentiation of disease and differentiation of the pattern is very important.

● Therapeutic methods:

This disease is mainly characterized by red spots over the skin, fever, joint pain, mucocutaneous and thoracic pleural damage, cough and wheezing, edema, chest oppression, palpitations, abdominal pain, bloody stool, and mental disturbances. This disease can affect the entire body. Any aspect, including the organs and connective tissue, can be damaged. The treatment should be focused on regulating the nutrient qi and defensive qi. Often this disease begins with symptoms of wind-dampness. Therefore, one should treat this disease as early as possible.

● Types and treatment:

1. The first type is marked by red spots over localized regions of skin, especially in the face, with an itching and burning feeling. Sometimes the red spots appear over the palms. This can be treated by clearing heat and removing toxin. The formulas used are *Yuè Bì Tāng* (Maidservant From Yue Decoction), *Má Xìng Shí Gān Tāng* (Ephedra, Apricot Kernel, Gypsum and Licorice Decoction), *Fáng Jǐ Dì Huáng Tāng* (Radix Stephaniae Tetrandrae and Radix Rehmanniae Decoction, 防己地黄汤), and *Gě Gēn Tāng* (Pueraria Decoction), modified, with the addition of *jīn yín huā* (Flos Lonicerae), *pú gōng yīng* (Herba Taraxaci), *lián qiào* (Fructus Forsythiae), and *dà qīng yè* (Folium Isatidis) in order to clear heat and remove toxin.

【 Case Study 】

Ren, male, had red spots all over his skin and was treated with the formulas mentioned above. After taking seven doses of the medicines, the red spots disappeared. When the patient stopped taking the medicine, the red spots appeared again. After further treatment, the red spots disappeared.

2. The second type manifests with albumen and red blood cells in the urine. At the advanced stage, the functions of the kidneys change, leading to uremia and nephritis. This type is due to both yang deficiency and yin deficiency.

[Pattern 1]

Yang deficiency with excess damp.

Though this disease mainly damages the kidney, it sometimes also affects the spleen and stomach. If spleen-yang declines, it will lead to sloppy stool, chest oppression, low appetite, and white and greasy tongue coating. In this case, the treatment should be focused on treating the spleen and stomach by warming and tonifying the spleen-yang. *Dì huáng* (Radix Rehmanniae) should not be used lest the spleen be damaged. Usually *Xiāng Shā Liù Jūn Zǐ Tāng* (Costusroot and Amomum Six Gentlemen Decoction) and *Wèi Líng Tāng* (stomach Calming Poria Decoction) are used. When spleen-yang is restored and the main symptoms have disappeared, the treatment should be focused on the kidney. If kidney-yang is weak, *Jīn Guì Shèn Qì Wán* (Golden Coffer Kedney Qi Pill) should be used with the addition of *dōng chóng xià cǎo* (Cordyceps), *yín yáng huò* (Herba Epimedii), *bā jǐ tiān* (Radix Morindae Officinalis) and *lù róng* (Cornu Cervi Pantotrichum). If there appear symptoms of scanty urine and body swelling, *Má Huáng Fù Zǐ Xì Xīn Tāng* (Ephedra, Aconite and Asarum Decoction) should be used with the addition of *chén xiāng* (Lignum

Aquilariae Resinatum), *ròu guì* (Cotex Cinnamomi), and *gān jiāng* (Rhizoma Zingiberis), in order to nourish the heart, promote urination, warm yang and transform water. If there is blood deficiency, the formula should be used with *Dāng Guī Bǔ Xuè Tāng* (Chinese Angelica blood Supplementing Decoction). If there is excessive urine protein, *huáng qí* (Radix Astragali) porridge should be taken. If there is insufficient protein in the blood and there is edema, carp soup should be taken. If the patient easily catches cold, *Yù Píng Fēng Sǎn* (Jade Wind-Barrier Powder) should be used.

〖 Case Study 〗

Zhao, male, 50 years old, was hospitalized in 1960 because of nephritis and uremia. Later on, he was diagnosed as suffering from lupus erythematosus. *Guì Fù Bā Wèi Tāng* (Cassia Bark and Aconite Eight Ingredient Decoction), *Dāng Guī Bǔ Xuè Tāng* (Chinese Angelica blood Supplementing Decoction) and *Chūn Zé Tāng* (Spring Pond Decoction) were used first to deal with the main pattern. At the same time the nutrient qi and defensive qi were also regulated to relieve the symptoms. After taking several hundred doses of the medicines, he gradually recovered.

[Pattern 2]

Yin deficiency with heat.

This type is characterized by reddish complexion, general weakness, rapid and forceful pulse, and a large amount of red blood cells in the urine. This should be treated by *Yuè Bì Tāng* (Maidservant From Yue Decoction), *Gě Gēn Tāng* (Pueraria Decoction), *Má Xìng Yì Gān Tāng* (Ephedra, Apricot Kernel, Coix, and Licorice Decoction, 麻杏薏甘汤), and *Fáng Jǐ Dì Huáng Tāng* (Radix Stephaniae Tetrandrae and Radix Rehmanniae Decoction), with the addition of herbs to clear heat and nourish yin, such as *Zhī Bǎi Dì Huáng Tāng* (Anemarrhena, Phellodendron and Rehmannia Decoction), *bái máo gēn* (Rhizoma Imperatae) and *guī jiǎ* (Carapax et Plastrum Testudinis).

【 Case Study 】

Li, male, suffered from albuminuria for a long time and later were diagnosed as lupus erythematosa. The manifestations were rapid and forceful pulse, red tongue, thirst and vexation. The main formula was used, with the addition of *Zhī Bǎi Dì Huáng Tāng* (Anemarrhena, Phellodendron and Rehmannia Decoction), *jīn yín huā* (Flos Lonicerae), *lián qiào* (Fructus Forsythiae), and *pú gōng yīng* (Herba Taraxaci).

[Pattern 3]

Heart type.

This type appears as rheumatic arthritis at the early stage. Later on, the symptoms of heart disease begin to appear. Sometimes it looks like coronary heart disease. Since the main symptoms are all related to the limbs and joints, the treatment should be focused on the limbs and joints first. If there is Painful Chest-Obstruction, *Guā Lóu Xiè Bái Bái Jiǔ Tāng* (Trichosanthes, Chinese Chive and White Wine Decoction) and *Fáng Jǐ Dì Huáng Tāng* (Radix Stephaniae Tetrandrae and Radix Rehmanniae Decoction) should be used with the addition of herbs to clear heat and remove toxin. Some cases can be treated by *Má Xìng Yì Gān Tāng* (Ephedra, Apricot Kernel, Coix, and Licorice Decoction, 麻杏薏甘汤). If there is hypertension, herbs such as *cǎo jué míng* (Semen Cassiae), *shēng dài zhě shí* (Haematitum), *gōu téng* (Ramulus Uncariae Cumuncis), *niú xī* (Radix Achyranthis Bidentatae), *shēng lóng gǔ* (Os Draconis), *shēng mǔ lì* (Concha Ostreae) and *yě jú huā* (Flos Chrysanthemi) should be added to the formula.

【 Case Study 】

Yu, female, 48 years old.In 1967, she began to run a fever at night. Later on, there appeared the symptoms of aching pain in the muscles, flaccidity, diffiulcty in walking, and low fever. In 1970, she was hospitalized because of high fever. After treatment with antibiotics, the fever still lingered. Then she was transferred to another hospital. Examination in that hospital found evidence of lupus erythematosus. After four months of treatment with Chinese medicine and modern medicine, her body temperature dropped to 37.5-38℃, her blood sedimentation dropped to 50mm/hour, but she was still unable to walk. In 1972, she came to me to receive treatment. Her manifestations then were heart and chest pain, aching and weakness of legs, dry mouth, difficulty in defecataion, weak pulse and atrophy of the legs. The formulas used were *Guā Lóu Xiè Bái Bái Jiǔ Tāng* (Trichosanthes, Chinese Chive and White Wine Decoction), *Dāng Guī Bǔ Xuè Tāng* (Chinese Angelica blood Supplementing Decoction) and *Guì Zhī Gān Cǎo Tāng* (Cinnamon Twig and Licorice Decoction, 桂枝甘草汤), with the addition of *yín yáng huò* (Herba Epimedii), *fú líng* (Poria), *gǒu qǐ zǐ* (Fructus Lycii), and *dǎng shēn* (Radix Codonopsis). After taking 30 doses of the medicines, the formula was used together with *Fáng Jǐ Dì Huáng Tāng* (Radix Stephaniae Tetrandrae and Radix Rehmanniae Decoction). One month later, *Hòu Jiāng Bàn Gān Shēn Tāng* (Officinal Magnolia Bark, Ginger, Rhizoma Pinelliae, Licorice, and Ginseng Decoction), with modifications, was added. Three months later, *wū shé ròu* (Black Snake Meat, 乌蛇肉) 30g and *qín jiāo* (Radix Gentianae Macrophyllae) 12g were added. Two months later, the original formula alone was used with modification. After one year of treatment, her arthralgia was significantly relieved and the patient could walk without a cane. In 1975, her arthritis disappeared. In 1976 her Painful Chest-Obstruction was basically cured. In March 1977, she began to take *Guā Lóu Xiè Bái Gě Gēn Tāng* (Fructus Trichosanthis, Bulbus Allii Macrostami and Radix Puerariae Decoction), which she continues to take.

[Pattern 4]

Gastrointestinal type.

This type is marked by vomiting, lumbago, hematemesis, bloody stool, poor appetite, and physical weakness. This type often occur or worsen in women during menstruation. It should be treated first by *Gān Cǎo Xiè Xīn Tāng* (Licorice heart Draining Decoction) for regulating the intestines and stomach, then by *Huáng Tǔ Tāng* (Yellow Earth Decoction) and *Chì Xiǎo Dòu Dāng Guī Sǎn* (Semen Phaseoli and Radix Angelicae Sinensis Powder, 赤小豆当归散) for stopping bleeding. When the symptoms of the digestive tract are relieved, bleeding will stop automatically and red spots will appear over the cheeks. If there is protein in the urine accompanied by sore-throat and oral ulceration, the main formulas, *Yuè Bì Tāng* (Maidservant From Yue Decoction), *Gě Gēn Tāng* (Pueraria Decoction), *Má Xìng Yì Gān Tāng* (Ephedra, Apricot Kernel, Coix, and Licorice Decoction), and *Fáng Jǐ Dì Huáng Tāng* (Radix Stephaniae Tetrandrae and Radix Rehmanniae Decoction), are used with the adddition of *Shān dòu gēn* (Radix Sophorae Tonkinensis), *bái máo gēn* (Rhizoma Imperatae) and *pú gōng yīng* (Herba Taraxaci). At the same time, *Xiè Xīn Tāng* (heart Draining Decoction) and *Huáng Tǔ Tāng* (Yellow Earth Decoction) are used alternatively.

〖 Case Study 〗

Zhou, female, adult.

Symptoms of gastrointestinal lupus erythematosus appeared. She was cured by the formulas mentioned above. The gastrointestinal bleeding during menstruation stopped. Her digestive functions were restored. The only sequela were red spots over the cheeks and mouth ulcers. Later on she was transferred to another hospital.

[Pattern 5]

Cerebral type.

This type of lupus erythematosus is caused by invasion of pathogenic factors into the brain, leading to the symptoms of auditory hallucination, visual hallucination, mental disturbance, high fever, talking to oneself, abnormal behavior and abnormal changes of cerebral spinal fluid. The formulas to be used are *Ān Gōng Niú Huáng Wán* (Peaceful Palace Bovine Bezoar Pill, 安宫牛黄丸) and *Zhì Bǎo Dān* (Supreme Jewel Elixir) for resuscitation and strengthening the heart, removing toxin and transforming turbidity in the blood with fragrant herbs. Herbs for expelling parasites can be used to regulate the nervous system.

【 Case Study 】

Liu, male, 60 years old.

He suffered from lupus erythematosa for years, which was worsened in recent months. The clinical manifestations were auditory hallucination, visual hallucination, mental disturbance, high fever, speaking to himself, abnormal behavior and abnormal changes of cerebral ans spinal fluid. The formula of *Gě Gēn Tāng* (Pueraria Decoction) was changed into *Gě Gēn Huáng Qín Huáng Lián Tāng* (Pueraria, Scutellaria, and Coptis Decoction), with the addition of two pills of *Zhì Bǎo Dān* (Supreme Jewel Elixir), plus *quán xiē* (Scorpio) and *wú gōng* (Scolopendra). After taking 4 doses of the medicines, his fever was relieved and his mental state was improved. Then *Ān Gōng Niú Huáng Wán* (Peaceful Palace Bovine Bezoar Pill) and *Zhì Bǎo Dān* (Supreme Jewel Elixir) were taken one pill each every day. After taking tens doses of the original formula, the condition of the patient was significantly improved. Then *Xiǎo Xiàn Xiōng Tāng* (Minor Chest Binding Decoction) and *Guā Lóu Xiè Bái Bàn Xià Tāng* (Trichosanthes, Chinese Chive and Pinellia Decoction) were used with the addition of other herbs for relieving spasm. For a time, the patient was better, but after one month of treatment, the disease of the patient worsened again, with delirium and abnormal body temperature. Then the formula for treating cerebral-type of lupus erythematosus was used together with Western medicine. This treatment did not take effect, and the patient eventually died. This case shows that cerebral type of lupus erythematosus, though critical, can still be effectively treated by Chinese herbs. If one can begin treatment early enough, the effect can be quite good. Biopsy showed that both kidneys were withered.

[Pattern 6]

liver type.

This type of lupus erythematosus is caused by invasion of pathogenic factors into the liver, marked by hepatomegaly, right hypochondriac pain, lack of appetite, unproductive vomiting, abdominal distension and abnormal changes of liver functions. The formulas to be used are *Sì Nì Sǎn* (Frigid Extremities Powder), *Xiǎo Chái Hú Tāng* (Minor Bupleurum Decoction) and *Chái Píng Tāng* (Bupleurum stomach-Calming Decoction, 柴平汤). I do not have much experience in treating this type of lupus erythematosus.

[Pattern 7]

Pulmonary type.

This type of lupus erythematosus is caused by invasion of pathogenic factors into the lung, marked by cough and wheezing, fever, night sweating, shortness of breath, weakness, lack of appetite, blood in the sputum and restless sleep. The formulas are *Má Xìng Shí Gān Tāng* (Ephedra, Apricot Kernel, Gypsum and Licorice Decoction), *Bǎi Hé Dì Huáng Tāng* (Bulbus Lilii Decoction and Radix Rehmanniae Decoction), *Bǎi Hé Zhī Mǔ Tāng* (Bulbus Lilii and Rhizoma Anemarrhenae Decoction) and *Mài Mén Dōng Tāng* (Radix Ophiopogonis Decoction), with the addition of herbs for removing toxin.

[Pattern 8]

Joint type.

This type of lupus erythematosus only affects the joints at the early stage. It can be treated by the main formula combined with *Xuān Bì Tāng* (Painful Obstruction Resolving Decoction), with modification, composed of *hǎi tóng pí* (Cortex Erythrinae), *piān jiāng huáng* (Rhizoma Curcumae Longae), *sāng jì shēng* (Herba Taxilli), *guì zhī* (Ramulus Cinnamomi), *bái sháo* (Radix Paeoniae Alba), *shēng dì* (Radix Rehmanniae), *yì yǐ rén* (Semen Coicis), *fáng jǐ* (Radix Stephaniae Tetrandrae), *xìng rén* (Semen Armeniacae Amarum), *cán shā* (Excrementum Bombycis), *zhī mǔ* (Rhizoma Anemarrhenae), *gān cǎo* (Radix Glycyrrhizae) and *má huáng* (Herba Ephedrae).

These eight types of lupus erythematosus are actually not completely separate from each other, and often appear together, but one type is usually predominant. Therefore, they should be treated according to pattern differentiation.

[Discussion]

1. Although there was no disease called lupus erythematosa in ancient times, there were similar diseases in the medical literature. "Wandering arthralgia recorded in *Jīn Guì Yào Lüè* (*Essential Prescriptions of the Golden Coffer*) is not lupus erythematosus, but is quite similar to rheumatic arthritis. It can be treated by *wū tóu* (Radix Aconiti) for dispersing cold, while at the same time regulating the nutrient qi and defensive qi. This is a similar idea to the treatment of the joint type of lupus. The disease known as *Ròu Jí* (extreme emaciation), recorded in *Jīn Guì Yào Lüè* (*Essential Prescriptions of the Golden Coffer*), has body fever with great loss of fluids, and open pores and interstices, severe wind qi, and lower *jiao* and leg weakness is quite similar to lupus. Also, in chapter five of the *Jīn Guì Yào Lüè* (*Essential Prescriptions of the Golden Coffer*), there is a disease characterized by mania, craziness, talking to oneself without stop, lack of fever of chills but with a floating pulse, that is similar to the cerebral type

of lupus erythematosus. It is treated with *Fáng Jǐ Dì Huáng Tāng* (Radix Stephaniae Tetrandrae and Radix Rehmanniae Decoction), which uses expel wind herbs for regulating the nutrient qi and defensive qi, together with blood-level herbs. This shows that this disease is located at the blood-level. These ideas are still useful today.

According to the classics of Chinese medicine and present clinical practice, nutrient qi and defensive qi play a very important role in the pathogenesis of this disease. The pathogenic obstruction of the nutrient qi and the defensive qi causes abnormal circulation in these energies. Since yang is not sufficient, then the defensive qi is damaged, which causes water to flow into the stomach instead of the spleen transporting to up to the lung and down to the bladder. Instead, the water overflows into the skin and muscles, which causes a pathological transformation in these areas. If yin is insufficient, the nutrient qi will be damaged and pathogenic factors will be retained in the body. Prolonged retention of pathogenic factors will transform into heat that scorches the nutrient qi and dessicates the muscles and blood. That is why the key for treating lupus erythematosus lies in regulation of the nutrient qi and defensive qi.

2. Blood vessesl are very important in treating lupus erythematosus. Doctors in the previous dynasties all paid great attention to the protection of blood vessels. This disease often occurs among women and becomes worsened during menstruation. In the clinical treatment of this disease in women, the practitioner must take blood vessels into careful consideration.

3. Based on the classics and my personal practice, I feel that the pathogenic factors of lupus erythematosus is located at the nutrient qi and defensive qi. When the nutrient qi and defensive qi are attacked, menses will become abnormal. So the treatment of this disease should be focused on regulating the nutrient qi and defensive qi, clearingheat andremoving toxin, cooling the blood to remove obstruction, and eliminating pathogenic factors and toxin. The formulas to be used are

Yuè Bì Tāng (Maidservant From Yue Decoction), *Gě Gēn Tāng* (Pueraria Decoction), *Má Xìng Yì Gān Tāng* (Ephedra, Apricot Kernel, Coix, and Licorice Decoction), and *Fáng Jǐ Dì Huáng Tāng* (Radix Stephaniae Tetrandrae and Radix Rehmanniae Decoction), with the addition of other ingredients. In *Yuè Bì Tāng* (Maidservant From Yue Decoction), *má huáng* (Herba Ephedrae) and *gān cǎo* (Radix Glycyrrhizae), sweet in taste and hot in nature, is used to regulate spleen-yang and remove pathogenic factors of yin nature; *shēng shí gāo* (Gypsum Fbrosum) and *gān cǎo* (Radix Glycyrrhizae), sweet in taste and cold in nature, is used to regulate stomach-yin and removing pathogenic factors of yang nature. In *Má Xìng Yì Gān Tāng* (Ephedra, Apricot Kernel, Coix, and Licorice Decoction), *má huáng* (Herba Ephedrae) enters the lung, and *xìng rén* (Semen Armeniacae Amarum) enters the heart, and are used to promote blood flow and, when combined with *yì yǐ rén* (Semen Coicis), eliminate stagnation and remove pathogenic factors from the muscles. *Gān cǎo* (Radix Glycyrrhizae) is used to relieve pain, strengthen the middle, remove toxin and subdue swelling. *Gě Gēn Tāng* (Pueraria Decoction) is used to dilate vessels, promote blood flow, expel pathogenic factors through sweating and remove toxin. It is stronger than *Guì Zhī Tāng* (Cinnamon Twig Decoction) in inducing sweating, and is often used to treat stiffness of the neck and back, aching pain of the body and joints, inflammation of the nose and mouth. *Fáng Jǐ Dì Huáng Tāng* (Radix Stephaniae Tetrandrae and Radix Rehmanniae Decoction) can disperse wind in the blood. *Shēng dì* (Radix Rehmanniae), sweet in taste and cold in nature, can remove wind-heat in the blood. Wind causes dryness. That is why herbs for cooling the blood must be used in dispersing wind, especially in dealing with cerebral type of lupus erythematosus, in which pathogenic factors have entered the Pericardium, pathogenic heat is in the blood and the heart-spirit is confused. In treating redness of the skin over the legs and hands or all over the body with burning pain caused by excessive taking of warm and dry herbs for treating Wind-Damp disease, Wang Xu-gao in the Qing Dynasty used *Fáng Jǐ Dì Huáng Tāng* (Radix Stephaniae Tetrandrae and Radix Rehmanniae Decoction). The curative effect was extraordinary. The four formulas mentioned above can be used with the addition of herbs for clearing heat to remove toxin, such as *pú gōng yīng* (Herba Taraxaci), *jīn yín huā* (Flos Lonicerae) and *shān dòu gēn* (Radix Sophorae Tonkinensis).

4. The immuno-suppressants in Western medicines used to treat lupus erythematosus may damage qi and blood. Corticosteroids may be effective for treating some patients, but it may also strengthen yang.

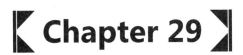

Chapter 29

Pathogenesis and Treatment of Skin Diseases

In traditional Chinese medicine, there are many methods for treating skin diseases. In recent years I have cured many patients with skin problems by regulating the nutrient qi and defensive qi and removing toxin. According to my personal experience, skin diseases are usually caused by a combination of the external and internal pathogenic factors. The most relevant external pathogens are wind, damp, dryness, and heat, but the internal factors of the seven abnormal emotions obstructing the normal functioning of the nutrient qi and defensive qi is the main cause of skin diseases.

Chinese medicine believes that human life depends on qi and blood. The functions of qi and blood are to nourish and defend the body. The function of the qi and blood is the nutritive and Defensice; the embodiment of the nutritive and the defensive is the qi and blood. When qi and blood flow smoothly, the nutrient qi and defensive qi will be in harmony and the body will be healthy. If the blood vessels become stagnant, diseases, including skin problems, will result. According to the theory of Chinese medicine, qi warms the body and blood nourishes the body. The book entiled *Zhù Jiě Shāng Hán Lùn* (Explanation of Treatise on Seasonal Febrile Diseases, 注解伤寒论) says: "*Cold body is due to failure of defensive qi to warm the body; hardness of the skin is due to failure of the nutrient qi to moisten the body.*" This shows that there is a close relationship between the qi and blood, the nutrient qi and defensive qi, and skin disease. It is well know from ancient times that the nutrient qi flows inside the vessels while the defensive qi flows outside the vessels. According to the *Huáng Dì Nèi Jīng* (Yellow Emperor's Inner Canon) and the *Shāng Hán Lùn* (Treatise on Seasonal Febrile Diseases), outside the vessels there is warm skin and muscles that are nourished by qi and blood. Therefore, the nutrient qi must flow outside of the vessles, together with the defensive qi. Although the nutrient qi mainly flows inside the vessels, and the defensive qi mainly flows outside of the vessels, both exit and enter and flow throughout the body and cannot be separated.

Just as yin and yang depend on each other, the nutrient qi and defensive qi also rely on each other for existence. That is what the phrase, "Qi is the commander of the blood" means. The blood is the essence of the five *zang* organs. If the five *zang* organs are in disharmony, the nutrient qi will decline. If the nutrient qi has declined, it will be unable to nourish the muscles, resulting in an imbalance between the nutrient qi and defensive qi. A disharmony between the nutrient qi and defensive qi can be adjusted by herbs. Clinically, the treatment is focused on regulating the nutrient qi and defensive qi and removing toxin. According to the *Jīn Guì Yào Lüè (Essential Prescriptions of the Golden Coffer)*, *Pái Nóng Sǎn* (Pus-Expelling Powder, 排脓散) is composed of *zhǐ shí* (Fructus Aurantii Immaturus), *sháo yào* (Chinese herbaceoous peony), *jié gěng* (Radix Platycodi) and *jī zǐ huáng* (Vitellus Galli); *Pái Nóng Tāng* (Pus-Expelling Decoction) is composed of *gān cǎo* (Radix Glycyrrhizae), *jié gěng* (Radix Platycodi), *shēng jiāng* (Rhizoma Zingiberis Recens) and *dà zǎo* (Fructus Jujubae). These herbs are all effective for promoting qi flow, activating the blood, and regulating the nutrient qi and defensive qi. Other formulas to be used are *Yuè Bì Tāng* (Maidservant From Yue Decoction), *Má Xìng Yì Gān Tāng* (Ephedra, Apricot Kernel, Coix, and Licorice Decoction), *Gě Gēn Tāng* (Pueraria Decoction), *Fáng Jǐ Dì Huáng Tāng* (Radix Stephaniae Tetrandrae and Radix Rehmanniae Decoction), *Xuān Bì Tāng* (Painful Obstruction Resolving Decoction), *Xiè Xīn Tāng* (heart Draining Decoction), *Jīng Fáng Bài Dú Sǎn* (Schizonepeta and Saposhnikovia Toxin Resolving Powder, 荆防败毒散), *Shēng Jiàng Sǎn* (Ascending and Descending Powder, 升降散), and *Dú Huó Jì Shēng Tāng* (Pubescent Angelica and Mistletoe Decoction, 独活寄生汤).

● Therapeutic methods:

1. For treating seborrheic dermatitis and senile pruritus, the formula is composed of:

Chinese Name	Pin Yin	Amount	Latin Name
防风	*fáng fēng*	9g	Radix Saposhnikoviae
苍术	*cāng zhú*	12g	Rhizoma Atractylodis
桑枝	*sāng zhī*	24g	Ramulus Mori
浮萍	*fú píng*	12g	Herba Spirodelae
茵陈蒿	*yīn chén hāo*	18g	Herba Artemisiae Scopariae
薏苡仁	*yì yǐ rén*	30g	Semen Coicis
地肤子	*dì fū zǐ*	18g	Fructus Kochiae
猪苓	*zhū líng*	12g	Polyporus
金银花	*jīn yín huā*	30g	Flos Lonicerae
地丁	*dì dīng*	9g	Herba Violae
皂角刺	*zào jiǎo cì*	6g	Spina Gleditsiae

2. For treating neurodermatitis and universal eczema, the formua to be used is composed of:

Chinese Name	Pin Yin	Amount	Latin Name
桂枝	*guì zhī*	9g	Ramulus Cinnamomi
麻黄	*má huáng*	6g	Herba Ephedrae
葛根	*gé gēn*	18g	Radix Puerariae
生石膏	*shēng shí gāo*	18g	Gypsum Fbrosum
甘草	*gān cǎo*	9g	Radix Glycyrrhizae
薏苡仁	*yì yǐ rén*	18g	Semen Coicis
杏仁	*xìng rén*	9g	Semen Armeniacae Amarum
白芍	*bái sháo*	9g	Radix Paeoniae Alba
当归尾	*dāng guī wěi*	12g	Radix Angelicae Sinensis
大黄	*dà huáng*	3g	Radix et Rhizoma Rhei
生姜	*shēng jiāng*	9g	Rhizoma Zingiberis Recens
大枣	*dà zǎo*	7 pieces	Fructus Jujubae

For treating universal eczema, *cāng zhú* (Rhizoma Atractylodis) 15g and *huáng bǎi* (Cortex Phellodendri) 12g are added; for treating swollen legs, *Jī Míng Sǎn* (Cockcrow Powder, 鸡鸣散) is added.

3. For treating psoriasis, the formula to be used is composed of:

Chinese Name	Pin Yin	Amount	Latin Name
白蒺藜	bái jí lí	30g	Fructus Tribuli
苦参	kǔ shēn	12g	Radix Sophorae Flavescentis
皂角刺	zào jiǎo cì	12g	Spina Gleditsiae
蝉蜕	chán tuì	12g	Periostracum Cicadae
生石膏	shēng shí gāo	18g	Gypsum Fbrosum
麻黄	má huáng	6g	Herba Ephedrae
甘草	gān cǎo	9g	Radix Glycyrrhizae
薏苡仁	yì yǐ rén	18g	Semen Coicis
杏仁	xìng rén	9g	Semen Armeniacae Amarum
桂枝	guì zhī	9g	Ramulus Cinnamomi
白芍	bái sháo	9g	Radix Paeoniae Alba
葛根	gé gēn	18g	Radix Puerariae
当归尾	dāng guī wěi	12g	Radix Angelicae Sinensis
大黄	dà huáng	3g	Radix et Rhizoma Rhei
生姜	shēng jiāng	9g	Rhizoma Zingiberis Recens
大枣	dà zǎo	7 pieces	Fructus Jujubae
海桐皮	hǎi tóng pí	18g	Cortex Erythrinae
白鲜皮	bái xiān pí	18g	Cortex Dictamni

〖 Chapter 30 〗

Treatment of Threatened Miscarriage and Functional Uterine Bleeding With Modified *Huáng Tǔ Tāng* (Yellow Earth Decoction)

According to the *Jīn Guì Yào Lüè* (Essential Prescriptions of the Golden Coffer), *Huáng Tǔ Tāng* (Yellow Earth Decoction, 黄土汤) treats distal bleeding. When yang enters yin, qi and the blood will be warmed and harmonized. When qi warms the body and blood nourishes the body, yin and yang will be well balanced. If qi is deficient, yang cannot command the blood and therefore cause uterine bleeding. If qi is excessive, it will produce fire and drive the blood to flow abnormally, causing hematemesis and nasal bleeding. If the blood is excessively lost, heat will also be discharged. That is why the six herbs in *Huáng Tǔ Tāng* (Yellow Earth Decoction) treat both qi and blood. These six herbs are *fù zǐ* (Radix Aconiti Lateralis Preparata), *bái zhú* (Rhizoma Atractylodis Macrocephalae), *gān cǎo* (Radix Glycyrrhizae), *dì huáng* (Radix Rehmanniae), *ē jiāo* (Colla Corii Asini), and *huáng qín* (Radix Scutellariae). Since heat and cold are equal, and since there is distal bleeding in the intestines, a heavy dosage of *huáng tǔ* (Terra Flava Usta) is used. In ancient times, threatened miscarriage and functional uterine bleeding were called "*bēng*, 崩", which means excessive uterine bleeding, like the collapse of a mountain, or the bottom of a bucket falling out. The cause of it is in the penetrating vessel and the *ren* vessel. The penetrating vessel and the *ren* vessel governs the *Tiān Guǐ* (reproductive substance/Heavenly Water, 天癸) and are different from the intestines that control defecation. Therefore, a heavy dosage of *shú dì huáng* (prepared Rhizome of Rehmannia, 熟地黄) and *lù jiǎo jiāo* (Colla Cornus Cervi) are used to tonify the penetrating vessel and the *ren* vessel. *Huáng tǔ* (Terra Flava Usta) is used to involve the girdling vessel.

Shēng dì huáng (unprepared Radix Rehmanniae, 生地黄) in ancient times refers to *xiān dì huáng* (fresh Radix Rehmanniae, 鲜地黄) in the present times. What is called *shēng dì huáng* (unprepared Radix Rehmanniae) now is known as *gān dì huáng* (dry Radix Rehmanniae, 干地黄) in ancient times. The note about *Bǎi Hé Dì Huáng Tāng* (Bulbus Lilii and Radix Rehmanniae Decoction) in the book entitled *Běn Jīng* (本经)

that "the stool is as black as lacquer" shows that *shēng dì huáng* (Radix Rehmanniae) can promote blood flow. Chen Nian-zu (陈念祖) in the Qing Dynasty said: "*Shú dì huáng* (prepared Rhizome of Rehmannia) is sticky greasy in nature, just as mixing flour with oil. It cannot be used if there are remaining pathogenic factors." I have used *Huáng Tǔ Tāng* (Yellow Earth Decoction) to stop uterine bleeding. Such a treatment makes use of the sticky and greasy properties of *shú dì* (prepared Rhizome of Rehmannia). The dosage of *shú dì* (Radix Rehmanniae) can be up to 60g. Tang Zong-hai (唐宗海) in the Qing Dynasty said that an upward flow of blood should be treated by descending therapy, while a downward flow of blood should be treated by ascending therapy. *Lù jiǎo jiāo* (Colla Cornus Cervi), ascending in nature and tonifying the Governor vessel, can be used to treat uterine bleeding. *é jiāo* (Colla Corii Asini), suppressing in nature and tonifying the *ren* vessel, can be used to treat hematemesis and epistaxis.

[Formula]

Chinese Name	Pin Yin	Amount	Latin Name
熟地黄	*shú dì huáng*	60g	Radix Rehmanniae Praeparata
龙眼肉	*lóng yǎn ròu*	30g	Arillus Longan
当归	*dāng guī*	12g	Radix Angelicae Sinensis
黄芪	*huáng qí*	18g	Radix Astragali
白术	*bái zhú*	9g	Rhizoma Atractylodis Macrocephalae
附子	*fù zǐ*	9g	Radix Aconiti Lateralis Preparata
甘草	*gān cǎo*	9g	Radix Glycyrrhizae
黄芩	*huáng qín*	9g	Radix Scutellariae
鹿角胶	*lù jiǎo jiāo*	30g	Colla Cornus Cervi
伏龙肝	*fú lóng gān*	12g	Terra Flava Usta

These ten ingredients are decocted in twelve cups of water. *Fú lóng gān* (Terra Flava Usta) is decocted first into eight cups of decoction. When the dregs are removed, the other eight ingredients are put in it to decoct.

When these dregs are removed, *lù jiǎo jiāo* (Colla Cornus Cervi) is melted and put into the decoction.

〖 Case Studys 〗

[Case 1]

Zhao, female, my neighbour, was pregnant for the first time after marriage. She suffered from dripping uterine bleeding threatened miscarriage in the early stage of pregnancy. After careful deliberation, I prescribed several doses of modified *Huáng Tǔ Tāng* (Yellow Earth Decoction). After taking the medicines, she was cured and later on gave birth to a baby girl. During her second pregnancy, she again had sign of a threatened miscarriage. I again prescribed several doses of the previous formula for her and she eventually gave birth to another baby girl.

[Case 2]

Cheng suffered from a miscarriage when she was pregnant for the first time. When she was pregnant for the second time, she had signs of a threatened miscarriage. I prescribed several doses of modified *Huáng Tǔ Tāng* (Yellow Earth Decoction). Her husband worked in a hospital and took my prescription to the hospital to buy the herbs. When doctors in that hospital saw *fù zǐ* (Radix Aconiti Lateralis Preparata) in the prescription, they thought it was a herb for inducing abortion and refused to give it to her husband. I advised her husband to buy it by himself. After taking the medicines prescribed, she was cured and eventually gave birth to a baby girl.

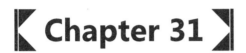

〖 Chapter 31 〗

Treatment of Auditory Vertigo (Meniere Disease)

CHAPTER 31　TREATMENT OF AUDITORY VERTIGO (MENIERE DISEASE)........223

Inner ear vertigo, also known as Meniere disease, is a kind of sudden vertigo, accompanied by nausea, vomiting, tinnitus, sensation of the room spinning, and fainting. This disease is commonly encountered in clinical practice. In traditional Chinese medicine it is called *Fēng Xuàn* (Wind Dizziness, 风眩). There are different ideas about the treatment of this disease. The therapeutic methods suggested are calming the liver to eliminate wind, nourishing yin to tonify the kidney, replenishing essence to enrich the Marrow and supplementing qi to nourish the blood. Clinical experience has proved that it can be treated by warming yang and draining water.

There are many records about the treatment of this disease in ancient literature. Liu He-jian treated vertigo from the aspect of wind while Zhu Dan-xi (朱丹溪) dealt with it from the aspect of phlegm. Luo Guo-gang (罗国纲) treated it from the aspect of the kidney, according to the idea that "deficiency in the upper causes vertigo; deficiency of the Governor vessel causes heaviness and tremor of the head," and "brain and marrow insufficiency, then there is ear ringing and dizziness," as described in the *Huáng Dì Nèi Jīng* (Yellow Emperor's Inner Canon). The *Huáng Dì Nèi Jīng* (Yellow Emperor's Inner Canon) also says that, "All kinds of wind patterns and vertigo are related to the liver." So I treat vertigo from the aspect of the liver. There are two kinds of vertigo, one is marked by heaviness of the head and darkness before the eyes, the other is marked by swirling of the earth and the sky. What Luo Guo-gang treated is in fact the first kind of vertigo. That is why he focused on the deficiency aspect. What Liu He-jian and Zhu Dan-xi treated is actually the second kind of vertigo. That is why they focused on the aspect of wind and phlegm. Zou Run-an (邹润安) in the Qing Dynasty divided diseases caused by wind into three kinds: those that immediately occur after contracting an external pathogen, as in Cold Damage or Warm Diseases; the stubborn disease caused by invasion of wind into the qi and the blood, such as wind-dizziness and wind patterns involving the head and face caused by invasion of wind into the upper part of the body; and Intestinal wind patterns and stomach wind patterns caused by invasion of wind into the lower part of the body.

The vertigo in this disease is caused by obstruction of water and fluid inside the body and yang transforming into wind, not directly by wind and phlegm. The *Sù Wèn* (Plain Questions) says: "When water enters the stomach, it flows together with essence and is transferred to the spleen. The spleen distributes the essence to the lung to regulate water passage. The water is then transmitted to the bladder and spread to all the parts of the body." When the spleen and stomach are abnormal in transportation and transformation, the stomach cannot transfer the essence and therefore it will accumulate into phlegm. When the stomach fails to transport water, it will coagulate into thin fluids, making it difficult for the clear yang to ascend and turbid yin to descend. If the stomach fails to maintain its normal descending activity, vomiting will result. So if water is well treated, the vertigo will heal automatically. Early in the Eastern Han Dynasty, Zhang Zhong-jing developed practical therapeutic methods for treating vertigo, such as warming yang and draining water. The formulas used are *Zé Xiè Tāng* (Rhizoma Alismatis Decoction, 泽泻汤) and *Líng Guì Zhū Gān Tāng* (Poria, Cinnamon Twig, Atractylodes Macrocephala and Licorice Decoction), often used with modification. The herbs used are:

Chinese Name	Pin Yin	Amount	Latin Name
生龙骨	*shēng lóng gǔ*	18g	Os Draconis
牡蛎	*mǔ lì*	18g	Concha Ostreae
桂枝	*guì zhī*	9g	Ramulus Cinnamomi
白术	*bái zhú*	12g	Rhizoma Atractylodis Macrocephalae
甘草	*gān cǎo*	9g	Radix Glycyrrhizae
半夏	*bàn xià*	12g	Rhizoma Pinelliae
生姜	*shēng jiāng*	9g	Rhizoma Zingiberis Recens
云苓	*yún líng*	18g	Poria
陈皮	*chén pí*	12g	Pericarpium Citri Reticulatae
泽泻	*zé xiè*	18g	Rhizoma Alismatis

This treatment is focused on warming yang to eliminate water, strengthening the spleen and draining water. That is why it can reduce water and stop wind. In the formula, *fú líng* (Poria) is used to draining water. *Guì zhī* (Ramulus Cinnamomi), acrid in taste and warm in nature, is used to promote yang. The combined use of these two herbs can warm yang to transform water. *Bái zhú* (Rhizoma Atractylodis Macrocephalae) is used to strengthen the spleen and dry dampness. *Gān cǎo* (Radix Glycyrrhizae) is used to harmonize the middle and invigorate qi. The combined use of these two herbs can tonify the spleen to control water. *Bàn xià* (Rhizoma Pinelliae), *shēng jiāng* (Rhizoma Zingiberis Recens), and *chén pí* (Pericarpium Citri Reticulatae) are used to regulate the stomach to stop vomiting. *Zé xiè* (Rhizoma Alismatis) is used to guide water to flow downwards. *lóng gǔ* (Os Draconis) and *mǔ lì* (Concha Ostreae) are used to suppress yang.

〖 Case Study 〗

Shi, male, 39 years old, office worker.

He suffered from vertigo for over 10 years and recuperated in a hospital for two years. The diagnosis then was neurasthenia, so he stayed at home to rest for three years. After that he had vertigo every year for 1-2 months and his vomiting was aggravated. Before he came to our hospital, he went to *Xuanwu* Hospital in Beijing to examine his nerve system. The examination found nothing abnormal. Then he came to our hospital to receive treatment. The clinical manifestations were severe vertigo, dizziness, vomiting, lack of appetite, numbness of the hands and feet, tinnitus, blood pressure being 130/80mmHg, wiry and thin pulse, white tongue coating and tooth-marked tongue. The modern medical diagnosis was Meniere disease. Pattern differentiation showed that his problem was caused by upward flow water and failure of liver-yang to control water. *Zé Xiè Tāng* (Rhizoma Alismatis Decoction) and *Líng Guì Zhū Gān Tāng* (Poria,

Cinnamon Twig, Atractylodes Macrocephala and Licorice Decoction) were used with modification for warming yang and draining water.

[Formula]

Chinese Name	Pin Yin	Amount	Latin Name
云苓	*yún líng*	15g	Poria
白术	*bái zhú*	12g	Rhizoma Atractylodis Macrocephalae
桂枝	*guì zhī*	9g	Ramulus Cinnamomi
甘草	*gān cǎo*	9g	Radix Glycyrrhizae
生龙骨	*shēng lóng gǔ*	30g	Os Draconis (to be decocted first)
泽泻	*zé xiè*	15g	Rhizoma Alismatis
生姜	*shēng jiāng*	6g	Rhizoma Zingiberis Recens
大枣	*dà zǎo*	5 pieces	Fructus Jujubae
生牡蛎	*shēng mǔ lì*	30g	Concha Ostreae (to be decocted first)
陈皮	*chén pí*	9g	Pericarpium Citri Reticulatae
半夏	*bàn xià*	12g	Rhizoma Pinelliae
钩藤	*gōu téng*	12g	Ramulus Uncariae Cumuncis

After taking seven doses of the medicines, the dizziness and nausea were significantly improved. The patient only felt body pain and weakness. Seven doses of the formula were prescribed again with the addition of herbs for expelling wind and dredging the collaterals, such as *fáng jǐ* (Radix Stephaniae Tetrandrae) and *qín jiāo* (Radix Gentianae Macrophyllae). One month later, the symptoms of vertigo and nausea appeared again, but were more mild than before. I prescribed another ten doses of the previous formula for him. After taking the medicines, he was cured.

Vertigo in Meniere's pattern is actually not caused by wind and phlegm, but by internal obstruction of water and transformation of yang into wind. That is why the treatment should be focused on warming yang, removing fluid obstruction, strengthening the spleen, and draining water.

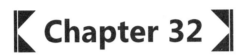

【 Chapter 32 】

Treatment of Arthritis

Arthritis pertains to the concepts of Bi-Pattern (pattern of blockage or obstruction, 痹症) and *Lì Jié Fēng* (swelling and pain of the joints, 历节风) in Chinese medicine. The bones are governed by the kidney and lubricated by the blood that is controlled by the heart. The tendons and ligaments are controlled by the liver while the muscles and joints are controlled by the spleen. So the joints are connected with the kidney, the liver, the spleen and the heart and are the places where visceral qi converges. The *Jīn Guì Yào Lüè* (Essential Prescriptions of the Golden Coffer) describes some kinds of wind Bi-Pattern and cold Bi-Pattern as *Lì Jié* that means that the joints are leaking and dripping. Such a description vividly shows the severity of this disease. Bi-Pattern refers to swelling and pain of joints due to stagnation of the vessels and channels caused by an invasion of exogenous pathogenic factors into the muscles, channels, and joints due to weakness of yang and deficiency of the exterior. It is now understood that this disease is caused wind, cold and dampness. We believe that this disease is actually caused by four pathogenic factors: wind, cold, dampness, and heat. In fact, some kinds of Bi-Pattern are mainly caused by pathogenic heat. It would be inaccurate to say that the heat in these kinds of Bi-Pattern is the heat transformed from stagnation of wind and cold.

Clinically, some kinds of Bi-Pattern are characterized by wind, some by dampness, some by cold, and some by heat. So the treatment principles should be decided according to the pathogenic factors involved. The treatment should be based on disease differentiation and pattern differentiation. There are eight therapeutic methods for treating Bi-Sydrome: expelling wind to discharge pathogenic factors, drying dampness to resolve dampness, warming yang to disperse cold, dredging the channels to smooth the collaterals, activating the blood to stop pain, supplementing qi to nourish the blood, nourishing the kidney to soften the tendons. Clinically, several methods may be used together according to pattern differentiation. If there is blood deficiency due to a prolonged duration of the disease, the method for invigorating qi and nourishing the blood should be used to eliminate wind; if there is blood stagnation, the methods for activating the blood to promote blood flow should be used; if there is cold, the methods for warming yang should be used, cold will be expelled when yang is invigorated; for draining dampness, the methods for strengthening spleen yang should be used, since dampness will be removed when yang is strengthened.

Some types of this disease pertain to connective tissue disorders in modern medicine because the organs of the patient are obviously changed and many of the organs are affected. Acute Wind-Damp diseases that tend towards a heat pathogenare categorized according to defensive-level, nutrient-level, qi-level and blood-level, and may invade the blood and affect the heart. About half of the related cases are children.

Chinese medicine divides Bi-Pattern into two categories, active stage and inactive stage. The latter is further divided inito rheumatic arthritis and rheumatoid arthritis. Rheumatic arthritis can be divided into four types: wind Bi-Pattern, cold Bi-Pattern, damp Bi-Pattern and heat Bi-Pattern. Rheumatoid arthritis pertains to the concepts of *Lì Jié* (swelling and pain of joints) and *Shèn Bì* (deformity of the bones, 肾痹).

Active Stage

Bi-Pattern at this stage includes wind Bi-Pattern and heat Bi-Pattern. Wind Bi-Pattern refers to migratory Bi-Pattern. Heat Bi-Pattern refers to redness, swelling, and pain of the joints, with the symptoms of fever, aversion to wind, and excessive thirst. Vessel Bi-Pattern described in the *Sù Wèn* (Plain Questions) pertains to heat Bi-Pattern because it is marked by burning pain of the skin, red patches over the skin, and irregular fever. This disease enters the nutritive and blood. If it is severe, it may manifest as heart Bi-Pattern, which involves the five *zang* organs. The methods used to treat it at the early stage are expelling wind to discharge pathogenic factors, clear heat to remove toxin, dredging the channels to smooth the collaterals, and activating the blood to dissipate stagnation. Then the methods for drying dampness and draining dampness are used.

[Formula]

Chinese Name	Pin Yin	Latin Name
秦艽	*qín jiāo*	Radix Gentianae Macrophyllae
连翘	*lián qiào*	Fructus Forsythiae
板蓝根	*bǎn lán gēn*	Radix Isatidis
蒲公英	*pú gōng yīng*	Herba Taraxaci
姜黄	*jiāng huáng*	Rhizoma Curcumae Longae
桑枝	*sāng zhī*	Ramulus Mori
生地	*shēng dì*	Radix Rehmanniae
蚕砂	*cán shā*	Excrementum Bombycis

Medicines for killing parasites can be added to eliminate wind, dredge the collaterals and adjust the nerves, such as *bái huā shé* (Agkistrodom, 白花蛇), *dì lóng* (Pheretima), and *jiāng cán* (Bombyx Batryticatus, 僵蚕). *Xī Líng Jiě Dú Wán* (Rhinoceros Horn and Antelope Horn Toxin Resolving Pill, 犀羚解毒丸) also can be added for removing toxin. If dampness is excessive, *Yuè Bì Tāng* (Maidservant From Yue Decoction) and *Má Xìng Yì Gān Tāng* (Ephedra, Apricot Kernel, Coix, and Licorice Decoction) can be used with modifications and the addition of *jīn yín huā* (Flos Lonicerae), *bǎn lán gēn* (Radix Isatidis), *zǐ cǎo* (Radix Arnebiae seu Lithospermi), *dān shēn* (Radix Salviae Miltiorrhizae) and *bái máo gēn* (Rhizoma Imperatae). If the disease affects the heart (manifested as palpitations, panting, dry throat, vexation and restlessness), *xī jiǎo* (Cornu Rhinocerotis Asiatici, *shuǐ niú jiǎo* or Cornu Bubali is now used, 水牛角), *dān pí* (Cortex Moutan Radicis), and *Zǐ Xuě Dān* (Purple Snow Elixir, 紫雪丹) can be added. If cerebral disease has occurred, *Ān Gōng Niú Huáng Wán* (Peaceful Palace Bovine Bezoar Pill, 安宫牛黄丸) can be added. If heat Bi-Pattern has deepened into the blood and changed into vessel Bi-Pattern with the symptoms of circular red spots over the skin, buring pain in the skin, rapid blood sedimentation and fever, it should be treated by clearing heat to cool the blood. The formula to be used is *Fáng Jǐ Dì Huáng Tāng* (Radix Stephaniae Tetrandrae and Radix Rehmanniae Decoction), *Xī Jiǎo Dì Huáng Tāng* (Rhinoceros Horn and Rehmannia Decoction, 犀角地黄汤) or *Huà Bān Tāng* (Macule-Transforming Decoction, 化斑汤) with the addition of *qīng dài* (Indigo Naturalis), *dì gǔ pí* (Cortex Lycii), *pú gōng yīng* (Herba Taraxaci), *jīn yín huā* (Flos Lonicerae), *lián qiào* (Fructus Forsythiae), and *qín jiāo* (Radix Gentianae Macrophyllae).

Inactive Stage

• Rheumatic arthritis:

1. Excessive pathogenic wind (Wind Bi-Pattern): This is characterized by wandering pain or aversion to wind, and should be treated by expelling wind to discharge the pathogenic factors and drying dampness and resolving dampness. The formula to be used is *Xuān Bì Tāng* (Painful Obstruction Resolving Decoction) with the addition of other ingredients. If there is heat, herbs for clearing heat and cooling the blood should be used. The formulas are *Yuè Bì Tāng* (Maidservant From Yue Decoction) and *Má Xìng Yì Gān Tāng* (Ephedra, Apricot Kernel, Coix, and Licorice Decoction) with modification. If there appears cold, the formula for warming yang and dispersing cold should be used, such as *Guì Zhī Sháo Yào Zhī Mǔ Tāng* (Cinnamon Twig, Peony and Rhizoma Anemarrhenae Decoction) with the addition of *dāng guī* (Radix Angelicae Sinensis), *fáng jǐ* (Radix Stephaniae

Tetrandrae), *wēi líng xiān* (Radix Clematidis, 威灵仙), *jiāng cán* (Bombyx Batryticatus), *dì lóng* (Pheretima), *shēng jiāng* (Rhizoma Zingiberis Recens) and *huáng qí* (Radix Astragali). Wind qi penetrated the liver, since the liver is the organ related to wind. The Bi-Pattern due to excessive wind should be treated by herbs for softening the tendons and dredging the liver, such as *bā jǐ tiān* (Radix Morindae Officinalis), *dù zhòng* (Cortex Eucommiae), *niú xī* (Radix Achyranthis Bidentatae), *sāng jì shēng* (Herba Taxilli), *ròu cōng róng* (Herba Cistanches), *bái sháo* (Radix Paeoniae Alba) and *cì jí lí* (Fructus Tribuli).

2. Excessive pathogenic cold (called Cold Bi-Pattern or Painful Bi-Pattern): This is characterized by sharp pain and inflexibility of joints, swollen feet, fixed pain that is alleviated with warmth and worsened with cold. It should be treated by the methods of warming yang and dispersing cold, dredging the channels and smoothing the collaterals, as well as activating the blood to stop pain. The formula to be used is *Guì Zhī Sháo Yào Zhī Mǔ Tāng* (Cinnamon Twig, Peony and Rhizoma Anemarrhenae Decoction). If it is severe, *Wū Tóu Guì Zhī Tāng* (Radix Aconiti and Ramulus Cinnamomi Decoction) can be used with the addition of *dāng guī* (Radix Angelicae Sinensis) and *huáng qí* (Radix Astragali). If there is blood deficiency and weakness of the body, it should be treated by invigorating qi and nourishing the blood. The formulas to be used are *Dāng Guī Shēng Jiāng Yang Ròu Tāng* (Radix Angelicae Sinensis, Rhizoma Zingiberis Recens and Mutton Decoction) and *Dāng Guī Bǔ Xuè Tāng* (Chinese Angelica blood Supplementing Decoction).

3. Excessive pathogenic dampness (also called Damp Bi-Pattern or Stagnation Bi-Pattern): This is characterized by heaviness of the limbs, fixated pain, inflexibility of the joints, difficulty turning turning the body, numbness of the muscles, and a white, thick, and greasy tongue coating. It is caused by spleen and kidney yang deficiency. The treatment should be focused on drying dampness, transforming dampness, warming yang, and

dredging the collaterals. The formulas to be used are *Gān Cǎo Fù Zǐ Tāng* (Radix Glycyrrhizae and Radix Aconiti Lateralis Preparata Decoction, 甘草附子汤) or *Má Huáng Fù Zǐ Xì Xīn Tāng* (Ephedra, Aconite and Asarum Decoction) and *Bái Zhú Fù Zǐ Tāng* (Rhizoma Atractylodis Macrocephalae and Radix Aconiti Lateralis Preparata, 白术附子汤).

Excessive water reduces fire. Excessive dampness weakens yang. That is why the methods for removing dampness and warming yang are used simultaneously. Only when the spleen is strengthened can dampness be removed. That is why heavy dosages of *fú líng* (Poria), *bái zhú* (Rhizoma Atractylodis Macrocephalae), and *fù zǐ* (Aconiti Lateralis Preparata) are used. If it lingers for a long time, heart failure and edema will appear. Then it should be treated by warming yang, eliminating cold, invigorating qi and nourishing the blood. In this case, *Zhēn Wǔ Tāng* (True Warrior Decoction) is used with the addition of *dāng guī* (Radix Angelicae Sinensis). If palpitations and a knotted and intermittent pulse appears, *Huáng Qí Wǔ Wù Tāng* (Radix Astragali Decoction Composed of Five Ingredients) and *Zhì Gān Cǎo Tāng* (Honey-Fried Licorice Decoction) should be used with the addition of *fú líng* (Poria) and *bái zhú* (Rhizoma Atractylodis Macrocephalae).

● Rheumatic arthritis, also known as Li Jie (swelling and pain of joints) or kidney Bi-Pattern:

This kind of Bi-Pattern is caused by a decline of yang, kidney deficiency, blood deficiency, liver and tendons lose nourishment, and invasion of exogenous wind. The joins are painful, swollen, and deformed. This should be treated by nourishing the blood, invigorating qi, nourishing the kidney, softening the tendons, eliminating wind, and warming yang. The methods to be used are eliminating dampness and activating the blood. If the blood is deficient, sweat cannot be produced. Therefore, it should be treated by the method of nourishing the blood to enrich the source of sweat. If only sweating therapy is used, the blood will be exhausted. Profuse sweating also exhausts yang. If both yin and yang are damaged, then it is difficult to treat this disease. Tonifying the kidney is exerted on the bones and soothing the liver is exerted on the tendons. Only when the methods for warming yang, removing wind, eliminating dampness, and activating the blood are used can it be effectively treated. The formula to be used is *Xiāo Shuǐ Shèng Yù Tāng* (Reduce Water to Sagely Cure Decoction); or *Guì Zhī Sháo Yào Zhī Mǔ Tāng* (Cinnamon Twig, Peony and Rhizoma Anemarrhenae Decoction) with the addition of *lù róng* (Cornu Cervi Pantotrichum), *bā jǐ tiān* (Radix Morindae Officinalis), *fáng jǐ* (Radix Stephaniae Tetrandrae), *dān shēn* (Radix Salviae Miltiorrhizae), *dù zhòng* (Cortex Eucommiae), *xù duàn* (Radix Dipsaci), and *niú xī* (Radix Achyranthis Bidentatae); or modified *Dāng Guī Shēng Jiāng Yáng Ròu Tāng* (Radix Angelicae Sinensis, Rhizoma Zingiberis Recens and Mutton Decoction). It can also be treated by *Wēi Shèn Wán* (Pill for Roasting the kidney, 煨肾丸).

There are some folk remedies that can also be tried. A part of fresh *sān qī* (Radix Notoginseng) leaf is decocted with brown sugar two or three times. The hot decoction is poured into the bowl with two eggs broken into it. This egg soup is taken orally over two days. When this remedy is taken, it will produce a slight sweat (the patient should take care to protect themselves from wind). This remedy treats chronic rheumatic arthritis.

[Formula Compositions]

Xiāo Shuǐ Shèng Yù Tāng (Reduce Water to Sagely Cure Decoction, 消水圣愈汤):

Chinese Name	Pin Yin	Latin Name
桂枝	*guì zhī*	Ramulus Cinnamomi
甘草	*gān cǎo*	Radix Glycyrrhizae
大枣	*dà zǎo*	Fructus Jujubae

Chinese Name	Pin Yin	Latin Name
姜	*jiāng*	Ginger
麻黄	*má huáng*	Herba Ephedrae
附子	*fù zǐ*	Radix Aconiti Lateralis Preparata
细辛	*xì xīn*	Herba Asari
知母	*zhī mǔ*	Rhizoma Anemarrhenae

Modified *Dāng Guī Shēng Jiāng Yáng Ròu Tāng* (Radix Angelicae Sinensis, Rhizoma Zingiberis Recens and Mutton Decoction, 当归生姜羊肉汤):

Chinese Name	Pin Yin	Amount	Latin Name
党参	*dǎng shēn*	15g	Radix Codonopsis
黄芪	*huáng qí*	30g	Radix Astragali
当归	*dāng guī*	30g	Radix Angelicae Sinensis
生姜	*shēng jiāng*	15g	Rhizoma Zingiberis Recens
羊肉	*yáng ròu*	250g	Mutton
桂枝	*guì zhī*	9g	Ramulus Cinnamomi
白芍	*bái sháo*	9g	Radix Paeoniae Alba

Wēi Shèn Wán (Pill for Roasting the kidney, 煨肾丸):

Chinese Name	Pin Yin	Latin Name
菟丝子	*tù sī zǐ*	Semen Cuscutae
草薢	*bì xiè*	Rhizoma Dioscoreae Hypoglaucae
肉苁蓉	*ròu cōng róng*	Herba Cistanches
杜仲	*dù zhòng*	Cortex Eucommiae
牛膝	*niú xī*	Radix Achyranthis Bidentatae
防风	*fáng fēng*	Radix Saposhnikoviae
白蒺藜	*bái jí lí*	Fructus Tribuli
桂枝	*guì zhī*	Ramulus Cinnamomi
胡芦巴	*hú lú bā*	Semen Trigonellae
补骨脂	*bǔ gǔ zhī*	Fructus Psoraleae
猪腰子	*zhū yāo zi*	Pig kidney

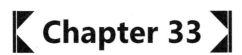

〖 Chapter 33 〗

Comments on *Hú Huò* (Behcet's Syndrome)

Hú Huò (erosion of mouth, eye, and genitalia) is a disease in Chinese medicine, similar to mouth-eye-genitals pattern in modern medicine. This disease is characterized by the simultaneous appearance of pustular inflammation of the iris and eyelid, ulceration and pain in the mouth, and ulcerations on the genitalia or anus. In 1937, H. Behcet, a Turkish dermatologist, discovered this disease in a patient, but this disease was recorded in the *Jīn Guì Yào Lüè* (Essential Prescriptions of the Golden Coffer). It can be treated by orally taking *Gān Cǎo Xiè Xīn Tāng* (Licorice heart Draining Decoction) and *Chì Xiǎo Dòu Dāng Guī Sǎn* (Semen Phaseoli and Radix Angelicae Sinensis Powder), along with external use *Kǔ Shēn Tāng* (Radix Sophorae Flavescentis Decoction, 苦参汤) and *Xióng Huáng Sǎn* (Realgar Powder) to wash the affected parts.

My years of clinical experience have proven that this disease is caused by the accumulation and steaming of damp-heat. According to the *Jīn Guì Yào Lüè* (Essential Prescriptions of the Golden Coffer), this disease can be treated by removing toxin and clearing damp-heat. The formula to be used is *Gān Cǎo Xiè Xīn Tāng* (Licorice heart Draining Decoction).

【 Case Study 】

Guo, female, 36 years old.

She suffered from oral and external genital ulcerations for half a year. At a hospital she was diagnosed as suffering from mouth-eye-genitals syndrome and treated her with hormones, but the effect was not satisfactory. I diagnosed her problem as *Hú Huò* (erosion of mouth, eye and genitalia), according to pulse differentiation. The formula used was *Gān Cǎo Xiè Xīn Tāng* (Licorice heart Draining Decoction) with the addition of other ingredients.

[Formula]

Chinese Name	Pin Yin	Amount	Latin Name
生甘草	*shēng gān cǎo*	30g	Radix Glycyrrhizae
党参	*dǎng shēn*	18g	Radix Codonopsis

Chinese Name	Pin Yin	Amount	Latin Name
生姜	*shēng jiāng*	6g	Rhizoma Zingiberis Recens
干姜	*gān jiāng*	3g	Rhizoma Zingiberis
半夏	*bàn xià*	12g	Rhizoma Pinelliae
黄连	*huáng lián*	6g	Rhizoma Coptidis
黄芩	*huáng qín*	9g	Radix Scutellariae
大枣	*dà zǎo*	7 pieces	Fructus Jujubae
生地	*shēng dì*	30g	Radix Rehmanniae

Twelve doses were prescribed. These ingredients were decocted in water for oral taking.

Four doses of *shēng gān cǎo* (Radix Glycyrrhizae) 12g and *kǔ shēn* (Radix Sophorae Flavescentis) 12g were prescribed. These two herbs were decocted and used to wash the external genitals. When she came for treatment the next time, her oral and genital ulcerations were already healed. Then I prescribed another fourteen dosese for oral taking and four does for washing. With this treatment, the patient was cured.

Index by Disease Names and Symptoms

A

aching pain in the muscles, 203
albuminuria, 203
alcoholic diarrhea, 132
anxiety due to deficiency of heart-yang, 175
arrhythmia, 052
asthma, 112
atrial fibrillation, 063
aversion to cold, 109
aversion to wind, 128

B

Bǎi Hé, 009, 168
barrel chest, 113
blockage of qi in the chest, 020
blood deficiency and damage of the fluids, 176
blood stagnation, 014
blood stasis, 073
blowing systolic murmur, 056
borborygmus, 128
bronchiectasis, 112
burning sensation during urination, 171

C

cardiac cirrhosis, 063
cerebral type, 205
chest oppression, 014, 024, 200
chest pain, 014
chest stuffiness, 110
chills, 144

choking when eating, 185
chronic bronchitis, 058
chronic cor pulmonale, 049, 058
chronic pneumocardial disease, 028
cold hernia, 192
cold invasion, 018
congestive heart failure, 050, 051
coronary atherosclerosis, 014
coronary heart disease, 016
cough, 018, 052, 102
cough in tuberculosis, 114
cough with purulent sputum, 114
counterflow cold, 002
cyanotic lips, 063

D

Da Jia Xie, 131
deficiency of both the heart and spleen, 174
deficiency of both the heart and the kidney, 048
deficiency of heart-yin and predominance of heart-Fire, 175
deficiency of heart yang, 015
diabetes, 082
diarrhea with indigested food in it, 128
diarrhea with indigestion, 135
diarrhea with poor appetite, 135
diarrhoea, 128

difficulty walking, 185
diffiulcty in walking, 203
distention of the jugular veins, 056
dizziness, 024, 197

E

edema, 048, 200
edema of the limbs, 058
encephalomalacia, 181
endogenous cough, 108
endogenous fever, 088
epigastric focal distention, 031, 122
erosion of the mouth, eye, and genitalia, 009
erythematosa, 208
excessive phlegm, 102
excessive sticky sputum, 058
exogenous cough, 108
exogenous fever, 088
extreme of the Flesh, 200

F

facial edema, 056
fatigue, 197
Fēng Xuàn, 224
feve, 079, 088, 144
feverish sensation over the palms and soles, 171
flaccidity, 203
floating and rapid pulse, 102
food diarrhea, 131
food epilepsy, 158

G

gastric ulcer, 089

gastrointestinal type, 204

greasy tongue coating, 234

H

heart failure, 031, 049, 058

heart type, 203

heaviness of the legs, 185

hepatomegaly, 048

high fever, 204

hoarse voice and rapid
breath, 028

Hú Huò, 009

hysteria, 169

I

inability to lie down, 053

infantile paralysis, 153

infantile pneumonia, 096

inflexibility of the right lower
limb, 185

insomnia, 018

insufficiency of kidney-yang,
197

insufficiency of yang in the
chest, 018

interior stirring of liver-Wind,
158

intermittent pulse, 021

internal and external heat,
104

J

joint pain, 200

Joint type, 207

K

kidney deficiency, 174

kidney diarrhea, 131

L

large intestine diarrhea, 130

Lì Fēng, 200

lily disease, 009, 168

lín zhèng, 078

liver diarrhea, 131

liver type, 207

loss of yang, 023

lower limb edema, 031, 056

low fever, 040

lumbago, 197

lupus erythematosus, 200

M

malaria, 142

male sterility, 196

Meniere disease, 224

Meniere's syndrome, 010

miscarriage, 222

mitral stenosis, 050

mucocutaneous and thoracic
pleural damage, 200

myocarditis, 036

N

nephritis, 068

neurasthenia, 174

numbness of the fingers, 178

O

obstruction of the vessels, 016

obstructive emphysema, 058

occasional tachycardia, 065

occasional vomiting, 018, 104

P

pain, 144

Painful Chest Obstruction,
014

pale complexion, 028

palpitations, 014, 040, 063

paroxysmal dyspnea, 054

pattern differentiation, 049

perceptual disturbances of
local areas in the limbs,
178

Pestilence Wind, 200

phlegm-dampness disturbing
the stomach, 176

phlegm-rheum epilepsy, 158

phlegm and dampness
stagnation, 053

phlegm diarrhea, 131

pleural effusion, 118

pneumonia, 096

Poliomyelitis, 148

poor appetite, 122

profuse sweating, 236

profuse sweating, 023

pulmonary blood stasis, 048

pulmonary type, 207

pustular inflammation, 240

pyelonephritis, 078

Q

Qi deficiency, 015

R

rapid, intermittent, and
knotted pulse, 036

red spots over the skin, 200

retention of phlegm and fluids, 029

rheumatic arthritis, 010

rheumatic heart disease, 063

Ròu Jí, 200

S

scanty urine, 058

severe angina pectoris, 016

severe chest and hypochondriac pain, 119

severe headache, 161

shaoyang diseases, 142

shaoyin disease, 007

shortness of breath, 014, 051, 063

slippery diarrhea, 129

sloppy diarrhea, 128

slurred speech, 185

small intestine diarrhea, 130

soggy diarrhea, 129

spasmodic cough, 110

spleen diarrhea, 130

spontaneous sweating, 051, 128

stagnation of lung qi, 049

stagnation of phlegm and dampness, 050

stomach diarrhea, 130

stomach distension, 054

stomach regurgitation, 015

subjective feeling of sudden mental confusion, 178

summer diarrhea, 132

superficial pathogenic heat, 086

superficial pattern, 086

swollen eyelids, 028

syphilis, 051

systolic murmur, 053

T

taiyang disease, 006

thin white greasy tongue coating, 028

tidal fever, 036, 039

tinnitus, 024

trigeminal neuralgia, 164

U

ulcerative disease, 122

upward counterflow of turbid qi of the stomach, 019

V

vertigo, 225

vertigo and headache, 185

vomiting of frothy white sputum, 052

W

warm disease, 100

weak pulse in the Cubit, 023

weak yang pulse, 015

Wind-Damp disease, 040

Wind-warm diseases, 096

wind Dizziness, 224

wind epilepsy, 158

wiry pulse, 128

wiry yin pulse, 015

worm epilepsy, 158

X

Xiǒng Bì, 014

Y

yang deficiency in the heart and kidney, 049, 050

yang deficiency with excess damp, 201

yangming diseases, 044

yellow sclera, 063

yin deficiency in the heart and lung, 051

yin deficiency with heat, 202

Index by Chinese Medicinals and Formulas

B

Bái Hǔ Jiā Guì Zhī Tāng, 143
bái máo gēn, 057
bái zhú, 002
bā jǐ tiān, 189
Bàn Xià Hòu Pò Tāng, 168
Bā Wèi Wán, 134
Bā Zhèng Sǎn, 078
Bì xie, 151
Blue Green Dragon
    Decoction, 006
bò he, 116
Bulbus Allii Macrostami, 019
Bǔ Yáng Huán Wǔ Tāng, 181

C

Cāng Zhú Bái Hǔ Tāng, 144
cǎo jué míng, 071
chái hú, 002
Chéng Qì Tāng, 003
chén xiāng, 072
Chinese Angelica blood
    Supplementing Decoction,
    021, 040, 204
chì sháo, 164
chì shí zhī, 123
Chlorite Phlegm Removing
    Pill, 159
Cinnamon Twig, Peony and
    Rhizoma Anemarrhenae
    Decoction, 010
Cinnamon Twig Decoction,
    002
Cinnamon Twig Decoction
    Plus Peony, 041
Coix Seed and Aconite

Powder, 022
Cornu Bubali, 232
Cortex Magnoliae Officinalis
    and Two Matured
    Substances Decoction, 131
Costus Root and Areca Pill,
    130

D

Dà Chéng Qì Tāng, 044
dāng guī, 193
Dāng Guī Bǔ Xuè Tāng, 021,
    040, 204
Dāng Guī Sháo Yào Sǎn, 073
Decoction for Cardiac Cough,
    113
Dì Fū Zǐ Tāng, 078
dì huáng, 189
Dì Huáng Yǐn Zǐ, 184
Dioscorea Pill, 076

E

Effective Integration
    Decoction, 124
Eight Ingredient Pill, 134
Ephedra, Aconite and
    Asarum Decoction, 108
Ephedra, Apricot Kernel,
    Coix, and Licorice
    Decoction, 202
Ephedra, Apricot Kernel,
    Gypsum and Licorice
    Decoction, 101, 200
Ephedra Decoction, 006
Èr Chén Tāng, 134
Exocarpium Citri Rubrum, 129

F

Fáng Jǐ Dì Huáng Tāng, 211
Fēng Yǐn Tāng, 158
Flos Inulae and Haematitum
    Decoction, 123
Four Pillar Drink, 129
Free Wanderer Powder, 090
Frigid Extremities Decoction,
    022, 089
Fructus Citri Reticulatae,
    Fructus Aurantii
    Immaturus, and Ginger
    Decoction, 020
Fructus Gleditsiae Pill, 018
Fructus Kochiae Decoction,
    078
Fructus Trichosanthis, 019
Fú Líng Xìng Rén Gān Cǎo
    Tāng, 021
fú lóng gān, 221
fù zǐ, 022

G

Galenite Elixir, 114
Gān Cǎo Xiè Xīn Tāng, 122, 240
Gān Mài Dà Zǎo Tāng, 169
gāo liáng jiāng, 128
Gě Gēn Huáng Qín Huáng
    Lián Tāng, 155
Ginseng and Perllia Beverage,
    115
Ginseng Toxin-Vanquishing
    Beverage, 161
Golden Coffer kidney Qi Pill,
    045
Gryllus Chinensis, 071

Grylotalpa Africana, 071

guā lóu, 019

Guā Lóu Xiè Bái Bàn Xià
Tāng, 019

guì zhī, 002

Guì Zhī Jiā Sháo Yào Tāng,
041

Guì Zhī Sháo Yào Zhī Mǔ
Tāng, 010

Guì Zhī Tāng, 002

Gypsum Fbrosum, 084

Gypsum Fibrosum, 029, 164

H

Halloysitum Rubrum, 123

Heart Draining Decoction,
003, 089

Hēi Xī Dān, 114

Herba Ephedrae, Fructus
Forsythiae and Semen
Phaseoli Decoction, 071

Herba Menthae, 116

Herba Taraxaci, 041

Hòu Pò Èr Chén Tāng, 131

Hòu Pò Má Huáng Tāng, 032,
058, 113

huáng qín, 125

Huáng Qín Huáng Lián Ē
Jiāo Jī Zǐ Huáng Tāng, 091

Huáng Qí Sháo Yào Tāng, 129

Huáng Qí Wǔ Wù Tāng, 235

Huáng Tǔ Tāng, 205

I

Immature Bitter Orange,
Chinese Chive and
Cinnamon Twig Decoction,
020

J

Jade Wind-Barrier Powder,
051

Jīn Gāng Wán, 148

Jīn Guì Shèn Qì Wán, 045

jú hóng, 129

Jú Zhǐ Jiāng Tāng, 020

K

Kidney-Qi Pill, 008

Kǔ Shēn Tāng, 240

L

Licorice, Wheat and Jujube
Decoction, 169

Licorice heart Draining
Decoction, 122, 240

Lignum Aquilariae
Resinatum, 072

Líng Guì Zhú Gān Tāng, 010

Liù Shén Wán, 075

Liù Zhù Yǐn, 130

Lǐ Zhōng Tāng, 129

lóu gū, 071

Lycium Berry,
Chrysanthemum and
Rehmannia Pill, 024

M

Má Huáng Fù Zǐ Xì Xīn Tāng,
108

Má Huáng Lián Qiào Chì
Xiǎo Dòu Tāng, 071

Maidservant From Yue
Decoction, 149, 200

Mài Mén Dōng Tāng, 111

Major Purgative Decoction,
044

Má Xìng Shí Gān Tāng, 101,
200

Má Xìng Yì Gān Tāng, 202

Méng Shí Gǔn Tán Wán, 159

Metal Strength Pill, 148

Middle Regulating Decoction,
129

Minor Blue Green Dragon
Decoction, 111, 159

Minor Bupleurum Decoction,
005

Minor Chest Binding
Decoction, 115

Minor Pinellia Decoction, 010

Mù Fáng Jǐ Tāng, 118

Mulberry Leaf and
Chrysanthemum Beverage,
103

mù xiāng, 128

Mù Xiāng Bīng Láng Wán,
130

Mù Xiāng Sǎn, 128

O

Officinal Magnolia Bark and
Ephedra Decoction, 032,
058, 113

P

Painful Obstruction
Resolving Decoction, 233

Pái Nóng Sǎn, 215

Pill for Roasting the kidney,
236

Pinellia and Officinal Magnolia Bark Decoction, 168

Polyporus Decoction, 079

Poria, Cinnamon Twig, Atractylodes Macrocephala and Licorice Decoction, 010

Poria, Semen Armeniacae Amarum and Radix Glycyrrhizae Decoction, 021

Pueraria, Scutellaria, and Coptis Decoction, 155

pú gōng yīng, 041

Pulse Engendering Powder, 030

Purgative Decoction, 003

Purple Snow Elixir, 138

Pus-Expelling Powder, 215

Q

Qǐ Jú Dì Huáng Wán, 024

Qīng Lóng Tāng, 006

R

Radix Aconiti and Ramulus Cinnamomi Decoction, 192

Radix Aconiti Lateralis Preparata, 022

Radix Angelicae Sinensis, 193

Radix Astragali Decoction Composed of Five Ingredients, 235

Radix Aucklandiae, 128

Radix Aucklandiae Powder, 128

Radix Bupleuri, 002

Radix Clematidis, 234

Radix glehniae, 116

Radix Glycyrrhizae Preparata, 125

Radix Morindae Officinalis, 189

Radix Ophiopogonis Decoction, 111

Radix Paeoniae Rubra, 164

Radix Rehmanniae, 189

Radix Scutellariae, 125

Radix Sophorae Flavescentis Decoction, 240

Radix Stephaniae Tetrandrae and Radix Rehmanniae Decoction, 211

Ramulus Cinnamomi, 002

Reduce Water to Sagely Cure Decoction, 029, 059

Rehmannia Drink, 184

Rén Shēn Bài Dú Yǐn, 161

Rescuing life Decoction, 178

Rhizoma Alismatis Decoction, 225

Rhizoma Alpiniae Officinarum, 128

Rhizoma Atractylodis Macrocephalae, 002

Rhizoma Dioscoreae Hypoglaucae, 151

Rhizoma Imperatae, 057

S

Sāng Jú Yǐn, 103

Semen Cassiae, 071

shā shēn, 116

Shēng dì huáng, 220

Shēng Mài Sǎn, 030

shēng shí gāo, 084

Shèn Qì Wán, 008

Shēn Sū Yǐn, 115

shí gāo, 029, 164

shuǐ niú jiǎo, 232

Shǔ Yù Wán, 076

Sì Nì Tāng, 022, 089

Six Pillar Drink, 130

Six Spirits Pill, 075

Sì Zhù Yǐn, 129

Sour Jujube Decoction, 020

Strengthening kidney yang and nourishing the kidney, 072

Suān Zǎo Rén Tāng, 020

T

Terra Flava Usta, 221

Tianxiong Aconite Powder, 196

Tiān Xióng Sǎn, 196

Trichosanthes, Chinese Chive and Pinellia Decoction, 019

True Warrior Decoction, 023, 030

Two Matured Substances Decoction, 134

U

unprepared Radix Rehmanniae, 220

W

wēi líng xiān, 234

Wēi Shèn Wán, 236

White Tiger Decoction
Composed of Rhizoma
Atractylodis, 144
White Tiger Plus Ramulus
Cinnamomi Decoction, 143
Wind-Eliminating Decoction,
158
Wū Tóu Guì Zhī Tāng, 192

X

Xiǎo Bàn Xià Tāng, 010
Xiǎo Chái Hú Tāng, 005
Xiǎo Qīng Lóng Tāng, 111, 159
Xiǎo Shuǐ Shèng Yù Tāng,
029, 059

Xiǎo Xiàn Xiōng Tāng, 115
Xiāo Yáo Sǎn, 090
xiè bái, 019
Xiè Xīn Tāng, 003, 089
Xīn Ké Tāng, 113, 116
xī shuài, 071
Xuān Bì Tāng, 233
Xù Mìng Tāng, 178

Y

Yang Supplementing and
Five Returning Decoction,
181
Yellow Earth Decoction, 205
Yī Guàn Jiān, 036, 124

Yì Yǐ Fù Zǐ Sǎn, 022
Yuè Bì Tāng, 031, 149, 200
Yù Píng Fēng Sǎn, 051

Z

Zào Jiǎ Wán, 018
Zēng Yè Tāng, 110
Zé Xiè Tāng, 225
Zhēn Wǔ Tāng, 023, 030, 061
zhì gān cǎo, 125
Zhǐ Shí Xiè Bái Guì Zhī Tāng,
020
Zhū Líng Tāng, 079
Zhú Yè Shí Gāo Tāng, 036
Zǐ Xuě Dān, 138

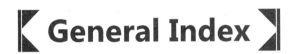

General Index

A

aching pain in the muscles,
203
activating the blood to stop
pain, 234
albuminuria, 203
alcoholic diarrhea, 132
anxiety due to deficiency of
heart-yang, 175
arrhythmia, 052
asthma, 112
astringe and bind, 134
astringing with sour herbs,
134
atrial fibrillation, 063
aversion to cold, 109
aversion to wind, 128

B

Bā jǐ tiān, 189
Bā Wèi Wán, 134
Bā Zhèng Sǎn, 078
Bǎi Hé, 009, 168
Bái Hǔ Guì Zhī Tāng, 143
bái máo gēn, 057
bái zhú, 002
Bàn Xià Hòu Pò Tāng, 168
barrel chest, 113
bì xiè, 151
bland elimination of
dampness, 133
blockage of lung qi, 057
blockage of qi in the chest,
020
blood deficiency and damage

of the fluids, 176
blood is the mother of the qi,
021
blood stagnation, 014
blood stasis, 073
blowing systolic murmur, 056
Blue Green Dragon
Decoction, 006
bò he, 116
borborygmus, 128
bronchiectasis, 112
Bǔ Yáng Huán Wǔ Tāng, 181
Bulbus Allii Macrostami, 019
burning sensation during
urination, 171

C

Cāng Zhú Bái Hǔ Tāng, 144
cǎo jué míng, 071
cardiac cirrhosis, 063
cerebral type, 205
chái hú, 002
chén xiāng, 072
Chéng Qì Tāng, 003
chest oppression, 014, 024,
200
chest pain, 014
chest qi, 016
chest stuffiness, 110
chì sháo, 164
chì shí zhī, 123
chills, 144
Chinese Angelica blood
Supplementing Decoction,
021, 040, 204
Chlorite Phlegm Removing

Pill, 159
choking when eating, 185
chronic bronchitis, 058
chronic cor pulmonale, 049,
058
chronic pneumocardial
disease, 028
Cinnamon Twig Decoction,
002
Cinnamon Twig Decoction
Plus Peony, 041
Cinnamon Twig, Peony and
Rhizoma Anemarrhenae
Decoction, 010
clearing and cooling, 133
clearing heat from the
nutrient level and
removing toxin, 099
clearing heat, releasing the
exterior, and expelling
phlegm, 118
Coix Seed and Aconite
Powder, 022
cold hernia, 192
cold invasion, 018
congestive heart failure, 050,
051
Cornu Bubali, 232
coronary atherosclerosis, 014
coronary heart disease, 016
Cortex Magnoliae Officinalis
and Two Matured
Substances Decoction, 131
Costus Root and Areca Pill,
130
cough, 018, 052, 102
cough in tuberculosis, 114

cough with purulent sputum, 114

counterflow cold, 002

cyanotic lips, 063

D

Dà Chéng Qì Tāng, 044

Da Jia Xie, 131

dāng guī, 193

Dāng Guī Bǔ Xuè Tāng, 021, 040, 204

Dāng Guī Sháo Yào Sǎn, 073

Decoction for Cardiac Cough, 113

defensive qi, 015

deficiency of both the heart and spleen, 174

deficiency of both the heart and the kidney, 048

deficiency of heart yang, 015

deficiency of heart-yin and predominance of heart-Fire, 175

Dì Fū Zǐ Tāng, 078

dì huáng, 189

Dì Huáng Yǐn Zǐ, 184

diabetes, 082

diarrhea with indigested food in it, 128

diarrhea with indigestion, 135

diarrhea with poor appetite, 135

diarrhoea, 128

difficulty walking, 185

diffiulcty in walking, 203

Dioscorea Pill, 076

disease differentiation, 002

distention of the jugular veins, 056

dizziness, 024, 197

drain water, 048

draining water, 118

dredging and draining, 133

dredging the channels and smoothing the collaterals, 234

drying the spleen, 134

E

edema, 048, 050, 200

edema of the limbs, 058

Effective Integration Decoction, 036, 124

Eight Ingredient Pill, 134

eliminate obstruction, 048

empting the urinary bladder, 048

encephalomalacia, 181

endogenous cough, 108

endogenous fever, 088

Ephedra Decoction, 006

Ephedra, Aconite and Asarum Decoction, 108

Ephedra, Apricot Kernel, Coix, and Licorice Decoction, 202

Ephedra, Apricot Kernel, Gypsum and Licorice Decoction, 101, 200

epigastric focal distention, 031, 122

Èr Chén Tāng, 134

erosion of mouth, eye and genitalia, 240

erosion of the mouth, eye, and genitalia, 009

erythematosa, 208

Essential Prescriptions of the Golden Coffer, 002

excessive phlegm, 102

excessive sticky sputum, 058

Exocarpium Citri Rubrum, 129

exogenous cough, 108

exogenous fever, 088

expelling pathogenic wind, 189

expelling wind and dredging the collaterals, 227

Explanation of Treatise on Seasonal Febrile Diseases, 214

Extreme of the Flesh, 200

F

facial edema, 056

Fáng Jǐ Dì Huáng Tāng, 211

fatigue, 197

Fēng Xuàn, 224

Fēng Yǐn Tāng, 158

fever, 079, 088, 144, 200

feverish sensation over the palms and soles, 171

five zang organs, 003

flaccidity, 203

floating and rapid pulse, 102

Flos Inulae and Haematitum

Decoction, 123

food diarrhea, 131

food epilepsy, 158

Four Pillar Drink, 129

Free Wanderer Powder, 090

Frigid Extremities Decoction, 022, 089

Fructus Citri Reticulatae, Fructus Aurantii Immaturus, and Ginger Decoction, 020

Fructus Gleditsiae Pill, 018

Fructus Kochiae Decoction, 078

Fructus Trichosanthis, 019

Fú Líng Xìng Rén Gān Cǎo Tāng, 021

fú lóng gān, 221

fù zǐ, 022

G

Galenite Elixir, 114

Gān Cǎo Xiè Xīn Tāng, 122, 240

Gān Mài Dà Zǎo Tāng, 169

gāo liáng jiāng, 128

gastric ulcer, 089

gastrointestinal type, 204

Gě Gēn Huáng Qín Huáng Lián Tāng, 155

Ginseng and Perllia Beverage, 115

Ginseng Toxin-Vanquishing Beverage, 161

Golden Coffer kidney Qi Pill, 045

Golden Mirror of Medicine, 009

greasy tongue coating, 234

Gryllus Chinensis, 071

Grylotalpa Africana, 071

guā lóu, 019

Guā Lóu Xiè Bái Bàn Xià Tāng, 019

guì zhī, 002

Guì Zhī Jiā Sháo Yào Tāng, 041

Guì Zhī Sháo Yào Zhī Mǔ Tāng, 010

Guì Zhī Tāng, 002

Gypsum Fibrosum, 029, 084, 164

H

Halloysitum Rubrum, 123

Heart Draining Decoction, 003, 089

heart failure, 031, 049, 058

heart type, 203

heaviness of the legs, 185

Hēi Xī Dān, 114

hepatomegaly, 048

Herba Ephedrae, Fructus Forsythiae and Semen Phaseoli Decoction, 071

Herba Menthae, 116

Herba Taraxaci, 041

high fever, 098, 204

hoarse voice and rapid breath, 028

Honey-Fried Licorice Decoction, 052

Hòu Pò Èr Chén Tāng, 131

Hòu Pò Má Huáng Tāng, 032, 058, 113

Hú Huò, 009, 240

Huáng Dì Nèi Jīng, 005

Huáng Qí Sháo Yào Tāng, 129

Huáng Qí Wǔ Wù Tāng, 235

huáng qín, 125

Huáng Qín Huáng Lián Ē Jiāo Jī Zǐ Huáng Tāng, 091

Huáng Tǔ Tāng, 205

hysteria, 169

I

imbalance between the nutrient qi and defensive qi, 215

Immature Bitter Orange, Chinese Chive and Cinnamon Twig Decoction, 020

Imperial Grace Pharmacy Formulas, 078

inability to lie down, 053

inducing sweating and removing toxin, 138

infantile paralysis, 153

infantile pneumonia, 096

inflexibility of the right lower limb, 185

insomnia, 018

insufficiency of kidney yang, 070, 197

insufficiency of yang in the chest, 018

interior stirring of liver-Wind,

158

intermittent pulse, 021

internal and external heat,
    104

invigorating qi, 062

J

Jade Wind-Barrier Powder,
    051

Jì Shēng Fāng, 078

Jīn Gāng Wán, 148

Jīn Guì Shèn Qì Wán, 045

Jīn Guì Yào Lüè, 002

joint pain, 200

Joint type, 207

jú hóng, 129

Jú Zhǐ Jiāng Tāng, 020

K

kidney controls urination and
    defecation, 135

kidney deficiency, 174

kidney diarrhea, 131

Kidney-Qi Pill, 008

Kǔ Shēn Tāng, 240

L

large intestine diarrhea, 130

Lì Fēng, 200

Lǐ Zhōng Tāng, 129

Licorice heart Draining
    Decoction, 122, 240

Licorice, Wheat and Jujube
    Decoction, 169

Life Saver Formulas, 078

Lignum Aquilariae

Resinatum), 072

lily disease, 009, 168

lín zhèng, 078

Líng Guì Zhú Gān Tāng, 010

Líng Shū, 014

Liù Shén Wán, 075

Liù Zhù Yǐn, 130

liver diarrhea, 131

liver type, 207

Lophatherum and Gypsum
    Decoction, 036

loss of yang, 023

lóu gū, 071

low fever, 040

lower limb edema, 031, 056

lumbago, 197

Lupus erythematosus, 200

Lycium Berry,
    Chrysanthemum and
    Rehmannia Pill, 024

M

Má Huáng Fù Zǐ Xì Xīn Tāng,
    108

Má Huáng Lián Qiào Chì
    Xiǎo Dòu Tāng, 071

Má Xìng Shí Gān Tāng, 101,
    200

Má Xìng Yì Gān Tāng, 202

Mài Mén Dōng Tāng, 111

Maidservant From Yue
    Decoction, 031

Maidservant From Yue
    Decoction, 149, 200

Major Purgative Decoction,
    044

malaria, 142

male sterility, 196

Méng Shí Gǔn Tán Wán, 159

Meniere disease, 224

Meniere's syndrome, 010

Metal Strength Pill, 148

Middle Regulating Decoction,
    129

Minor Blue Green Dragon
    Decoction, 111, 159

Minor Bupleurum Decoction,
    005

Minor Chest Binding
    Decoction, 115

Minor Pinellia Decoction, 010

miscarriage, 222

mitral stenosis, 050

Mù Fáng Jǐ Tāng, 118

mù xiāng, 128

Mù Xiāng Bīng Láng Wán,
    130

Mù Xiāng Sǎn, 128

mucocutaneous and thoracic
    pleural damage, 200

Mulberry Leaf and
    Chrysanthemum Beverage,
    103

myocarditis, 036

N

nephritis, 068

neurasthenia, 174

nourish qi and promote
    blood flow, 073

nourish the kidney and
    enrich the essence, 152

nourish yin, 038
nourishing both the heart and the spleen, 126
nourishing the heart, 062
nourishing yin and tonifying the qi, 082
nourishing yin to clear heat and reduce fire, 082
numbness of the fingers, 178
nutritive qi, 015

O

obstruction of the vessels, 016
obstructive emphysema, 058
occasional tachycardia, 065
occasional vomiting, 018, 104
Officinal Magnolia Bark and Ephedra Decoction, 032, 058, 113
On Cold Damage, 002
open yang, 038
opening the sweat pores, 048

P

Pái Nóng Sǎn, 215
pain, 144
Painful Chest Obstruction, 014
Painful Obstruction Resolving Decoction, 233
pale complexion, 028
palpitations, 014, 040, 063
paroxysmal dyspnea, 054
pattern differentiation, 002, 049
perceptual disturbances of

local areas in the limbs, 178
Pestilence Wind, 200
phlegm and dampness stagnation, 053
phlegm diarrhea, 131
Phlegm-dampness disturbing the stomach, 176
phlegm-rheum epilepsy, 158
Pill for Roasting the kidney, 236
Pinellia and Officinal Magnolia Bark Decoction, 168
Plain Questions, 014
pleural effusion, 118
pneumonia, 096
Poliomyelitis, 148
Polyporus Decoction, 079
poor appetite, 122
Poria, Cinnamon Twig, Atractylodes Macrocephala and Licorice Decoction, 010
Poria, Semen Armeniacae Amarum and Radix Glycyrrhizae Decoction, 021
profuse sweating, 023, 236
pú gōng yīng, 041
Pueraria, Scutellaria, and Coptis Decoction, 155
pulmonary blood stasis, 048
pulmonary type, 207
Pulse Engendering Powder, 030
Purgative Decoction, 003
Purple Snow Elixir, 138

Pus-Expelling Powder, 215
pustular inflammation, 240
pyelonephritis, 078

Q

qi deficiency, 015
qi is the commander of the blood, 021
Qǐ Jú Dì Huáng Wán, 024
Qīng Lóng Tāng, 006

R

Radix Aconiti and Ramulus Cinnamomi Decoction, 192
Radix Aconiti Lateralis Preparata, 022
Radix Angelicae Sinensis, 193
Radix Astragali Decoction Composed of Five Ingredients, 235
Radix Aucklandiae, 128
Radix Aucklandiae Powder, 128
Radix Bupleuri, 002
Radix Clematidis, 234
Radix glehniae, 116
Radix Glycyrrhizae Preparata, 125
Radix Morindae Officinalis, 189
Radix Ophiopogonis Decoction, 111
Radix Paeoniae Rubra, 164
Radix Rehmanniae, 189
Radix Scutellariae, 125
Radix Sophorae Flavescentis

Decoction, 240

Radix Stephaniae Tetrandrae
and Radix Rehmanniae
Decoction, 211

raising and lifting, 133

Ramulus Cinnamomi, 002

rapid, intermittent, and
knotted pulse, 036

red spots over the skin, 200

Reduce Water to Sagely Cure
Decoction, 029, 059

regulating the lung and the
stomach, 030

Rehmannia Drink, 184

release stagnant lung-qi, 109

remove stagnation and
invigorate yang, 019

remove toxin, 038

removing fluid retention, 158

Rén Shēn Bài Dú Yǐn, 161

Rescuing life Decoction, 178

resolving phlegm, 158

retention of phlegm and
fluids, 029

rheumatic arthritis, 010

rheumatic heart disease, 063

Rhizoma Alismatis
Decoction, 225

Rhizoma Alpiniae
Officinarum, 128

Rhizoma Atractylodis
Macrocephalae, 002

Rhizoma Dioscoreae
Hypoglaucae, 151

Rhizoma Imperatae, 057

Promoting production of
fluid, 083

Ròu Jí, 200

S

Sāng Jú Yǐn, 103

scanty urine, 058

Semen Cassiae, 071

severe angina pectoris, 016

severe chest and
hypochondriac pain, 119

severe headache, 161

shā shēn, 116

Shāng Hán Lùn, 002

shaoyang diseases, 142

shaoyin disease, 007

Shèn Qì Wán, 008

Shēn Sū Yǐn, 115

shēng dì huáng, 220

Shēng Mài Sǎn, 030

shēng shí gāo, 084

shí gāo, 029, 164

shortness of breath, 014, 051,
063

Shǔ Yù Wán, 076

shuǐ niú jiǎo, 232

Sì Nì Tāng, 022, 089

Sì Zhù Yǐn, 129

six *fu* organs, 003

Six Pillar Drink, 130

Six Spirits Pill, 075

slippery diarrhea, 129

sloppy diarrhea, 128

slurred speech, 185

Small intestine diarrhea, 130

soggy diarrhea, 129

Sour Jujube Decoction, 020

spasmodic cough, 110

Spiritual Pivot, 014

spleen and stomach yin
deficiency and fire, 082

spleen detests dampness and
likes dryness, 069

spleen diarrhea, 130

spontaneous sweating, 051,
128

stagnation of lung qi, 049

stagnation of phlegm and
dampness, 050, 056

stomach diarrhea, 130

stomach distension, 054

stomach regurgitation, 015

strengthen the heart yang, 048

strengthening kidney yang
and nourishing the kidney,
072

strengthening yang to
eliminate stagnation, 053

Sù Wèn, 014

Suān Zǎo Rén Tāng, 020

subjective feeling of sudden
mental confusion, 178

summer diarrhea, 132

summer-heat, 088

superficial pathogenic heat,
086

superficial pattern, 086

suppressing yang and
opening the collaterals, 179

swollen eyelids, 028

syphilis, 051

systolic murmur, 053

T

Tài Píng Huì Mín Hé Jì Jú
Fāng, 078

taiyang disease, 006

Terra Flava Usta, 221

thin white greasy tongue
coating, 028

Tiān Xióng Sǎn, 196

Tianxiong Aconite Powder,
196

tidal fever, 036, 039

tinnitus, 024

tonifying both the kidney
and the spleen, 196

transforming rheum and
eliminating phlegm, 159

Trichosanthes, Chinese Chive
and Pinellia Decoction, 019

Trigeminal neuralgia, 164

True Warrior Decoction, 023,
030

Two Matured Substances
Decoction, 134

U

ulcerative disease, 122

unprepared Radix
Rehmanniae, 220

upward counterflow of
turbid qi of the stomach,
019

V

vertigo, 225

vertigo and headache, 185

vomiting of frothy white
sputum, 052

W

warm disease, 100

warming and tonifying the
spleen yang, 069

warming the kidney, 134

warming yang, 057

warming yang and dispersing
cold, 234

warming yang, draining
water, transforming qi and
harmonizing the middle,
119

weak pulse in the Cubit, 023

weak yang pulse, 015

wēi líng xiān, 234

Wēi Shèn Wán, 236

White Tiger Decoction
Composed of Rhizoma
Atractylodis, 144

White Tiger Plus Ramulus
Cinnamomi Decoction, 143

wind Dizziness, 224

wind epilepsy, 158

Wind-Damp disease, 040

Wind-Eliminating Decoction,
158

wind-warm diseases, 096

wiry pulse, 128

wiry yin pulse, 015

worm epilepsy, 158

Wū Tóu Guì Zhī Tāng, 192

X

xī shuài, 071

Xiǎo Bàn Xià Tāng, 010

Xiǎo Chái Hú Tāng, 005

Xiǎo Qīng Lóng Tāng, 111,
159

Xiǎo Shuǐ Shèng Yù Tāng,
029, 059

Xiǎo Xiàn Xiōng Tāng, 115

Xiāo Yáo Sǎn, 090

xiè bái, 019

Xiè Xīn Tāng, 003, 089

Xīn Ké Tāng, 113, 116

Xiǒng Bì, 014

xū lǐ, 016

Xù Mìng Tāng, 178

Xuān Bì Tāng, 233

Y

yang deficiency in the heart
and kidney, 049, 050

Yang deficiency in the heart
and kidney, 056

Yang deficiency of the heart
and kidney, 031

Yang deficiency with excess
damp, 201

Yang Supplementing and
Five Returning Decoction,
181

yangming channel, 083

yangming diseases, 044

yellow and dry or light
yellow tongue coating, 098

Yellow Earth Decoction, 205

Yellow Emperor's Inner
Canon, 005

yellow sclera, 063

Yī Guàn Jiān, 036, 124

Yì Yǐ Fù Zǐ Sǎn, 022
Yī Zōng Jīn Jiàn, 009
yin deficiency in the heart
    and lung, 051
yin deficiency with heat, 202
Yù Píng Fēng Sǎn, 051
Yuè Bì Tāng, 031, 149, 200

Z

Zào Jiǎ Wán, 018
Zé Xiè Tāng, 225
Zēng Yè Tāng, 110
Zhang Zhong-jing, 004
Zhēn Wǔ Tāng, 023, 030, 061
zhì gān cǎo, 125

Zhì Gān Cǎo Tāng, 052
Zhǐ Shí Xiè Bái Guì Zhī Tāng,
    020
Zhù Jiě Shāng Hán Lùn, 214
Zhū Líng Tāng, 079
Zhú Yè Shí Gāo Tāng, 036
Zǐ Xuě Dān, 138

General Index·········263

图书在版编目（CIP）数据

赵锡武医疗经验（英文）/ 中国中医研究院西苑医院主编 .
—北京：人民卫生出版社，2008.6
（名老中医经验集系列）
ISBN 978-7-117-10225-4

Ⅰ . 赵… Ⅱ . 中… Ⅲ . 中医学临床—经验—中国—现代
Ⅳ . R249.7

中国版本图书馆 CIP 数据核字（2008）第 067323 号

赵锡武医疗经验（英文）

主　　编：中国中医研究院西苑医院
出版发行：人民卫生出版社（中继线 +8610-6761-6688）
地　　址：中国北京市丰台区方庄芳群园三区 3 号楼
邮　　编：100078
网　　址：http://www.pmph.com
E - mail：pmph @ pmph.com
发　　行：zzg@pmph.com.cn
购书热线：+8610-6769-1034（电话及传真）
开　　本：787×1092　1/16
版　　次：2008 年 6 月第 1 版　2008 年 6 月第 1 版第 1 次印刷
标准书号：ISBN 978-7-117-10225-4/R·10226